Immune
Responses
to
Metastases

Volume II

Editors

Ronald B. Herberman, M.D.
Director
Pittsburgh Cancer Institute
and
Professor of Medicine and Pathology
University of Pittsburgh
Pittsburgh, Pennsylvania

Robert H. Wiltrout, Ph.D.
Head
Experimental Therapeutics Section
Laboratory of Experimental
Immunology
Biological Response Modifiers Program
Division of Cancer Treatment
National Cancer Institute
Frederick, Maryland

Elieser Gorelik, M.D.
Investigator
Pittsburgh Cancer Institute
and
Associate Professor of Pathology
University of Pittsburgh
Pittsburgh, Pennsylvania

CRC Press, Inc.
Boca Raton, Florida

Library of Congress Cataloging-in-Publication Data

Immune responses to metastases.

   Includes bibliographies and index.
   1. Metastasis—Immunological aspects.
2. Immunotherapy. I. Herberman, Ronald B., 1940-
II. Wiltrout, Robert H. III. Gorelik, Elieser.
[DNLM: 1. Neoplasm Metastasis—immunology. 2. Neoplasm
Metastasis—therapy. QZ 202 I325]
RC268.3.I44 1987   616.99′4071   86-7878
ISBN 0-8493-5847-7 (v. 1)
ISBN 0-8493-5848-5 (v. 2)
ISBN 0-8493-5849-3 (set)

   Direct all inquiries to CRC Press, Inc., 2000 Corporate Blvd., N.W., Boca Raton, Florida, 33431.

© 1987 by CRC Press, Inc.

International Standard Book Number 0-8493-5847-7 (v. 1)
International Standard Book Number 0-8493-5848-5 (v. 2)
International Standard Book Number 0-8493-5849-3 (set)

Library of Congress Card Number 86-7878
Printed in the United States

PREFACE

The greatest limitation to the successful treatment of cancer is the ability of tumors to form distant metastases. These metastases are often located in vital organs and are either inaccessible or refractory to conventional forms of cancer treatment. In addition, primary tumors and their metastases are often composed of subpopulations or foci of tumor cells that differ in their sensitivity to the various forms of cancer treatment. This heterogeneity within a tumor cell population contributes appreciably to the inability of chemotherapeutic drugs or radiotherapy to completely eradicate established tumors and thereby cure rather than just delay the progression of the disease. A further limitation of conventional cancer treatment is the necessity to balance the toxicity of chemotherapy or irradiation for the patient with the dose-dependent beneficial antitumor effects of these modalities. Therefore, the ideal form of cancer therapy would be selective for the tumor and thereby nontoxic to the host, able to circumvent heterogeneity within a given tumor, and be able to reach tumor metastases in all anatomical sites. Based on these criteria, high expectations have arisen that the immune system can be explited as a weapon against cancer, and more specifically against metastases. The rationale for these high expectations is based on the exquisite specificity associated with T-lymphocytes and antibodies, the broad yet tumor selective cytotoxic activity of NK cells, LAK cells and macrophages, and the presence of these effector mechanisms in most organs and anatomical compartments. In order for immunologic approaches to the treatment of cancer to live up to their expected potential, it seems essential to systematically investigate the parameters required for optimal stimulation of effector activities and for selective accumulation of effector cells and/or molecules at the sites of metastases. This should provide the needed foundation for the rational design of therapeutic trials in experimental tumor systems and in patients with cancer.

In this volume, we have summarized the current status of the field and have attempted to identify major issues for future investigaitons. In particular, we have addressed three aspects of the relationship between the host immune system and tumor metastases. First, because the process of metastasis is complex, several chapters (Chapters 1 to 3) have been included to address various aspects of the metastatic phenotype which related to host-tumor interactions. These contributions summarize the evidence that considerable heterogeneity exists within metastatic tumor cell populations and illustrate the ways in which this heterogeneity influences, and is influenced by, the immune system. Secondly, the interaction between the immune system and metastases is bidirectional. Therefore, we have included contributions which are at least partially devoted to summarizing the impact of metastasis formation and tumor progression on various components of the immune system and the ways in which different parameters of immunity change in response to tumor growth (Chapters 1 to 7). Thirdly, and most central to the ultimate objective of this field or research, considerable attention is focused on approaches to modulating and utilizing host immunity for the express purpose of preventing or eradicating metastases (Chapter 8 to 14).

Overall, the chapters in this volume demonstrate that many advances have been made in understanding the metastatic process and host-tumor interactions. Further, significant advances have also been made with regard to modulation of immunity and our understanding of how to optimize this modulation. These insights already have translated into considerable progress in the development of successful strategies for the immunotherapy of experimental metastases. However, the successful application of these approaches to the treatment of human cancer remains to be developed. In the clinical trials with immunotherapy of metastases which are now being planned or are underway, it would seem important if not essential to follow the principles elucidated in these experimental systems, in order to optimize the potential of these approaches for the cure of human cancer.

THE EDITORS

Ronald B. Herberman, M.D., is Director of the Pittsburgh Cancer Institute and Professor of Medicine and Pathology at the University of Pittsburgh, Pennsylvania.

Dr. Herberman received his undergraduate and doctoral education at New York University, receiving a B.A. degree in 1960 and a M.D. degree in 1964. He then served as an intern and resident in internal medicine at the Massachusetts General Hospital from 1964 to 1966. He then went to the National Cancer Institute as a Clinical Associate in 1966 and then progressed to a series of positions of increasing responsibility, including Head of the Cellular and Tumor Immunology section of the Laboratory of Cell Biology, Chief of the Laboratory of Immunodiagnosis, and then Chief of the Biological Therapeutics Branch in the Biological Response Modifiers Program. In addition, during his last year at the National Cancer Institute he was Acting Associate Director for the Biological Response Modifiers Program. In 1985, he moved to Pittsburgh to begin the organization of a new cancer center, associated both with the University of Pittsburgh, Carnegie-Mellon University, and the University Health Center of Pittsburgh.

Dr. Herberman is a member of the American Association of Immunologists, American Association for Cancer Research, American Federation for Clinical Research, American Society for Clinical Investigation, Transplantation Society, and Reticuloendothelial Society. He is a Fellow of the American College of Physicians and of the American Academy of Microbiology. He was elected President of the Reticuloendothelial Society in 1984. He was awarded a commendation medal from the United States Public Health Service.

Dr. Herberman is the author of more than 600 papers and has been the Editor of six books. His current major research interests relate to cellular and tumor immunology and the use of immunological approaches for the diagnosis and therapy of cancer.

Robert H. Wiltrout, Ph.D., is Head of the Experimental Therapeutics Section at the Biological Response Modifiers Program of the National Cancer Institute's Frederick Cancer Research Facility, Frederick, Maryland. Dr. Wiltrout received his B.A. from Kutztown University, Kutztown, Pennsylvania, his M.S. from the Pennsylvania State University, University Park, Pennsylvania, and his Ph.D. from the Wayne State University School of Medicine, Detroit, Michigan.

Dr. Wiltrout is a member of several professional organizations, including the Reticuloendothelial Society, The American Association of Immunologists, and the Honorary Society Sigma Xi. He has published more than 90 articles, contributions to books, and abstracts. His current research interests include the biology of metastasis and the application of biological response modifiers to the treatment of cancer.

Elieser Gorelik, M.D., Ph.D. was born in the USSR. He graduated from the State Medical School, Minsk, USSR in 1961 and received his Ph.D. degree in 1968 from the Institute of Genetics and Cytology, Byelorussian Academy of Science. In 1975, he emigrated to Israel and worked at the Weizmann Institute of Science. In 1979, he was invited to come to the National Cancer Institute, National Institutes of Health, where he has worked until recently. He has just now initiated research at the Pittsburgh Cancer Institute. Dr. Gorelik is the author of about 100 articles, of which 70 were published after his emigration.

Dr. Gorelik is a member of several professional organizations, including the American Association for Cancer Research. His research interests relate to tumor immunology and investigation of the role of the immune system in the control of metastatic spread and growth.

CONTRIBUTORS

Paola Allavena, M.D.
Research Associate
Mario Negri Institute for
  Pharmacological Research
Milan, Italy

Peter Altevogt, Ph.D.
Associate Member
Institute Immunologie and Genetik
Deutsches Krebsforschungszentr
Heidelberg, West Germany

Malcolm George Baines, Ph.D.
Associate Professor
Department of Microbiology and
  Immunology
McGill University
Montreal, Quebec, Canada

Claudia Balotta, M.D.
Research Assistant
Mario Negri Institute for
  Pharmacological Research
Milan, Italy

Barbara Bottazzi, Ph.D.
Research Associate
Mario Negri Institute for
  Pharmacological Research
Milan, Italy

Jorge A. Carrasquillo, M.D.
Attending Physician
Department of Nuclear Medicine
National Institutes of Health
Bethesda, Maryland

Isaiah J. Fidler, D.V.M., Ph.D.
R. E. "Bob" Smith Chair in Cell
  Biology
Professor and Chairman
Department of Cell Biology
M.D. Anderson Hospital and Tumor
  Institute
Houston, Texas

William E. Fogler, Ph.D.
Research Scientist
Department of Membrane Biochemistry
Walter Reed Army Institute of
  Research
Washington, D.C.

Elieser Gorelik, M.D., Ph.D.
Investigator
Pittsburgh Cancer Institute
Associate Professor of Pathology
University of Pittsburgh
Pittsburgh, Pennsylvania

Michael G. Hanna, Jr., Ph.D.
Vice President and Director
Research and Development
Bionetics Research, Inc.
Rockville, Maryland

Nabil Hanna, Ph.D.
Director
Department of Immunology
Smith Kline and French Laboratories
Swedeland, Pennsylvania

Ruediger Heicappell, M.D.
Guest Scientist
Institute Immunologie and Genetik
Deutsches Krebsforschungszentrum
Heidelberg, West Germany

Ingegerd Hellström, M.D.
Vice President and Laboratory Director
Oncogene
University of Washington
Seattle, Washington

Karl Erik Hellström, M.D.
Vice President and Laboratory Director
Oncogene
University of Washington
Seattle, Washington

Gloria H. Heppner, Ph.D.
Scientific Director
Research Division
Michigan Cancer Foundation
Detroit, Michigan

Ronald B. Herberman, M.D.
Director
Pittsburgh Cancer Institute
and
Professor of Medicine and Pathology
University of Pittsburgh
Pittsburgh, Pennsylvania

Herbert C. Hoover, Jr., M.D.
Chief, Surgical Oncology
Division of Surgical Oncology
State University of New York, Stony
  Brook
Stony Brook, New York

Steven M. Larson, M.D.
Chief
Nuclear Medicine Department
National Institutes of Health
Bethesda, Maryland

Alberto Mantovani, M.D.
Chief
Laboratory of Human Immunology
Mario Negri Institute for
  Pharmacological Research
Milan, Italy

Fred R. Miller, Ph.D.
Associate Member
Department of Immunology
Research Division
Michigan Cancer Foundation
Detroit, Michigan

James J. Mulé, Ph.D.
Senior Staff Fellow
Surgery Branch
National Cancer Institute
National Institutes of Health
Bethesda, Maryland

David S. Nelson, D.Sc., F.R.A.C.P.
Director
Kolling Institute of Medical Research
The Royal North Shore Hospital of
  Sydney
St. Leonards, New South Wales,
  Australia

Garth L. Nicolson, Ph.D.
Florence M. Thomas Professor
  Cancer Research
Chairman
Department of Tumor Biology
University of Texas
M.D. Anderson Hosptial and Tumor
  Institute
Houston, Texas

Susan M. North, Ph.D.
Research Associate
Department of Tumor Biology
University of Texas
M.D. Anderson Hospital and Tumor
  Institute
Houston, Texas

Hugh F. Pross, M.D., Ph.D., F.R.C.P
Professor and Head
Department of Radiation Oncology,
  Microbiology, and Immunology
Queen's University
Kingston, Ontario, Canada

Steven A. Rosenberg, M.D., Ph.D.
Chief of Surgery
Surgery Branch
National Cancer Institute
National Institute of Health
Bethesda, Maryland

Volker Schirrmacher, Ph.D.
Head
Professor
Department of Cellular Immunology
Institute Immunologie and Genetik
Deutches Krebsforschungszentrum
Heidelberg, West Germany

James E. Talmadge
Head
Preclinical Screening Laboratory
Program Resources, Inc.
NCI-Frederick Cancer Research Facility
Frederick, Maryland

P. von Hoegen, Ph.D.
Student
Institute Immunologie and Genetik
Deutsches Krebsforschungzentru
Heidelberg, West Germany

Robert H. Wiltrout, Ph.D.
Head
Experimental Therapeutics Section
Laboratory of Experimental
 Immunology
Biological Response Modifiers Program
Division of Cancer Treatment
NCI-Frederick Cancer Research Facility
Frederick, Maryland

TABLE OF CONTENTS

VOLUME I

VOLUME II

Chapter 7

MODULATIONS OF TUMOR CELL IMMUNOGENICITY LEADING TO INCREASED T-CELL REACTIVITY AND DECREASED METASTASIS FORMATION

V. Schirrmacher, P. von Hoegen, R. Heicappell, and P. Altevogt

TABLE OF CONTENTS

I. INTRODUCTION

Previous studies with many chemically or virus induced animal tumors have shown that long lasting tumor immunity can be induced in syngeneic hosts against such immunogenic tumors by various immunization procedures. This effective antitumor immunity is based primarily on cellular immunity exerted by effector T-lymphocytes such as CTL, T-helper cells (T_H), and delayed type hypersensitivity T-cells (T_{DTH}). Unfortunately, when similar immunization protocols were applied for the treatment of human neoplasia the results have been disappointing. This has led to a serious criticism of the relevance of the animal model systems used, which were in most instances highly immunogenic and nonmetastatic tumors.

As a consequence of this situation, in recent years more experimental work has been performed with metastasizing animal tumors. Such tumors are often low or even non-immunogenic. It soon became apparent that the induction of protective immunity against such metastatic animal tumors was quite difficult to achieve. An additional problem arose when studies were performed with cloned lines of metastatic animal tumors. It turned out that such clones were not as stable as one had anticipated from the experience with nonmetastatic tumors. The instability of malignant tumor lines can lead to the generation of tumor heterogeneity and can thus play an important role in the process of tumor progression. These findings have serious implications for all types of tumor therapy because instability and variability of residual tumor mass could lead to the development of therapy resistant tumor variants. Immunotherapy for instance could be unsuccessful because of the development of immuno-resistant variants. Such considerations have influenced immuno-logical thinking towards the development of more unspecific modalities of immunological intervention, many examples of which are given in this book.

In spite of the mentioned problems of low immunogenicity and antigenic variability, we still believe in a potential role of specific cell mediated antitumor immune responses for the immunological intervention against cancer and its metastases. This attitude is based on new findings related to

1.   Generation of immunogenic variants by drug treatment.
2.   Reconstitution of tumor immunogenicity by gene transfer or gene activation.
3.   Modulations of tumor immunogenicity by virus xenogenization.

We will focus in the following mainly on these aspects and will discuss how this can lead to increased T-cell reactivity to metastatic tumor cells.

The hope that such approaches may eventually become applicable for antimetastatic immunotherapy is based on our steadily increasing knowledge about

1.   The immunobiology of metastasis.[1,2]
2.   Mechanisms of T-cell mediated antitumor immunity, its kinetics, regulation, and decay.[3-5]
3.   Culture conditions for growing effector T-lymphocytes to large quantities.[6]
4.   The use of immune T-cells for adoptive immunotherapy.[3,5,6]

II. T-CELL LYMPHOCYTE EFFECTOR RESPONSES TO SPONTANEOUS, APPARENTLY NONIMMUNOGENIC ANIMAL TUMORS

Naturally occurring animal tumors appear to be the more suitable models for comparison with human neoplasia than chemically or virus induced tumor lines. The question of immunogenicity of such spontaneous tumors is therefore of great importance and different views have been expressed.[7,8] According to the experience of Hewitt[7] naturally occurring tumors in rodents are unable to induce protective immunity in classical immunization-protection assays. This was interpreted as evidence for nonimmunogenicity.[7] However, the question remains whether negative results in immunization-protection assays really mean that such tumors are not recognized by the immune system. Would it not be possible that such tumors are recognized, but that the reponse is not sufficiently strong to lead to tumor rejection? As we will consider later also such nonimmunogenic tumors can be rendered immunogenic to a level detectable in classical immunization-protection assays. The question whether spontaneous tumors have the ability to trigger an immune reaction seems to be of fundamental importance because it will decide whether there is a "handle" for immunological intervention and manipulation.

In the following, immunogenicity will be defined in a rather broad sense as the ability of a tumor to trigger an immune reaction strong enough to affect tumor growth. As discussed in more detail elsewhere[9] this definition is not confined to the classical immunization-protection assays and includes mechanisms which can trigger specific and nonspecific host antitumor reactions.

Tumor cells may express antigenic deviations from corresponding normal cells which may result from those genetic changes which form the basis of the tumor development. Any antigenic deviation from normal on the part of neoplastic cells can provide the means for immunologic intervention and an important task of the immunologist would be to strengthen such weak tumor-associated antigens (TAA) and to transform them into potent immunogens.

An interesting example of a spontaneous mouse tumor with which the question of immunogenicity was studied in much detail using both in vivo and in vitro methods is the ADK-1t tumor investigated by Forni et al.[10] Although no resistance was observed in immunization-protection tests using various immunization schedules this tumor was found to affect the immune system of normal mice in various ways which influenced the tumor growth in vivo. The host responses following subcutaneous tumor implantation were characterized by spleen enlargement, increase of activated spleenic macrophages, appearance of antitumor cytotoxic T-lymphocytes (about 1 week after challenge) followed by suppressor activities in the serum (when the tumor reached a critical size). These host antitumor responses could be manipulated in a positive or negative way by either immunostimulation or by immunologic impairment leading to either decreased or increased tumor growth rate respectively.[9,10]

If spontaneous tumors can carry TAA structures recognizable by CTL, the question remains why no specific protective immunity can be detected. This question was recently investigated in a spontaneous rat fibrosarcoma tumor model.[11] This tumor, BSp6S, could not induce transplantation resistance but it could induce syngeneic CTL in vitro in the presence but not in the absence of IL-2. It was suggested that the TAA are not recognized by syngeneic helper T-cells (T_H) and that this may be the reason for lack of induction of protective immunity. In accordance with this hypothesis, it was shown that the lack of induction of T_H cells could be reconstituted by introducing new antigenic determinants (NAD) into the tumor cell surface.[11]

These experiments support the concept that cellular immune responses to cell surface antigens depend on the associative recognition of more than one antigenic determinant[12] in a similar way as immune responses to soluble hapten-carrier conjugates.[13] Activation of T_H for tumor specific CTL required physical association of NAD and TAA on the same cell thus enabling either intermolecular or intrastructural help.[12] Antigen presenting cells were probably also required for T_H cell activation since the tumor lacked class II major histocompatibility complex (MHC) antigens. The efficiency of antitumor immune responses in vivo was dependent on the presence of appropriately activated T_H.[11]

III. MODULATIONS OF TUMOR CELL IMMUNOGENICITY VIA MAJOR HISTOCOMPATIBILITY COMPLEX ANTIGENS

MHC antigens play an important role in the induction and regulation of cellular immune responses. CTL are known to recognize altered cell surface antigens on virus infected normal or on neoplastic cells as "foreign" when they are associated with class I MHC molecules.[14] Tumor cell recognition by CTL thus depends on the recognition of a TAA plus an MHC molecule. Lack of CTL recognition may thus be due to lack of either of these entities or at least to a reduced expression below the threshold of activation. One way in which tumor cells and in particular disseminating malignant cells may evade host defenses is by decreasing the expression of MHC class I genes whose products may serve as restricting elements. Some recent findings are consistent with this hypothesis:

1. There is an increasing number of reports showing lack of expression of certain MHC antigens on animal tumors[15] as well as on human tumors.[16]
2. There may be a tendency that such lack of expression is more frequently seen in metastasis as compared to locally growing tumors suggesting a role in immune escape.
3. Reconstitution of immunogenicity has been achieved by H-2 gene transfection. Hui et al.[17] reported that restoration of H-2K^k expression by gene transfection led to reduced tumorigenicity of a nonmetastatic AKR mouse thymoma. Wallich et al.[18] recently reported the abrogation of metastatic properties of tumor cells by *de novo* expression of H-2K antigens following H-2 gene transfection. These results suggest that metastatic spread could be limited by an immune response regulated through MHC class I antigens and offers hope for potential therapeutic application if it was possible to induce those antigens. Interferons for example induce a marked increase in the surface expression of these molecules.

It must be pointed out, however, that suppression of MHC class I genes on tumor cells is not a universal characteristic. There are even reports to the opposite, namely that increases in MHC class I gene expression are associated with metastatic capacity.[19] An inverse relationship has been suggested between the requirement of either NK or T-cells for recognition of MHC molecules on target cells whcich could explain some of the controversial findings.[33] Furthermore, it has been suggested that certain MHC molecules (e.g., H-2D) might exert a suppressive influence while others (e.g. H-2K) would provide a helper stimulus. A hypothesis was put forward that tumorigenicity and metastatic spread was influenced by the ratio of H-2K to H-2D molecules on the tumor cell surface. Such attempts for a unifying explanation for the regulation of metastatic spread are probably oversimplifications but they offer hypotheses that are amenable to experimental tests.

IV. MODULATIONS OF TUMOR CELL IMMUNOGENICITY VIA GENE ACTIVATION BY DNA DEMETHYLATING DRUGS

Another approach to increased tumor immunogenicity was introduced by Boon et al.[20] who showed that it is possible to obtain immunogenic tumor variants by mutagen treatment in vitro. Such variants, which can arise with a high frequency fail to form tumors in syngeneic mice and have therefore been termed tum⁻ variants. Tum⁻ variants fail to grow in immunocompetent mice because they elicit a strong immune rejection response in vivo. They also induce a specific CTL response in vitro. Most tum⁻ variants, which could be produced in many different tumor systems, were shown to carry new variant specific transplantation antigens. Furthermore, it was found that tum⁻ variants are capable of eliciting a protective response against the original tumor cell. This was even observed with spontaneous tumors of Hewitt which elicit no immune rejection responses. For three such tumors it was observed that tum⁻ variants elicited a protection against their original tumor but not against the others.[21] The results indicated the presence of weak tumor-associated transplantation antigens on spontaneous mouse tumors and this finding could be confirmed on the level of induction of specific CTL responses. It was thus shown that by the use of immunogenic variants it is possible to direct the immune response to weak antigenic determinants on apparently non-immunogenic spontaneous animal tumors.

These findings raised a number of new interesting questions and attracted the interest of various tumor immunologists. Frost et al.[22] investigated the mechanism of high frequency variant induction and reported that similar tum⁻ variants could be obtained by a virtually nonmutagenic drug called 5-azacytidine, a strong DNA-hypomethylating agent. 5-azacytidine and ethylmethanesulfonate (EMS) were found to be equally and comparably effective or ineffective in inducing tum⁻ variants when testing three different highly tumorigenic mouse cell lines. Like mutagen induced tum⁻ variants those obtained after 5-azacytidine treatment generated usually a strong CTL response in vitro and could grow in immunosuppressed hosts. Since it is known that treatment of cells with 5-azacytidine can induce transcriptional activation of "silent" genes through a reduction of DNA 5-methylcytosine content it was hypothesized that the generation of tum⁻ variants at high frequency by mutagenic DNA alkylating drugs or 5-azacytidine was due to DNA hypomethylation leading to the activation and expression of genes coding for potential tumor antigens[22] or other cellular determinants important for tumor cell immunogenicity.

We were interested to find out whether a similar mechanism could account for the generation of variants which arose under physiological conditions, namely as immune escape variants. We found that the highly metastatic tumor ESb,[23] which carries a specific TAA, can generate (especially during metastasis in immunocompetent hosts) at high frequency TAA loss variants which play an important role in the escape of the tumor cells from specific T-cell mediated immunity.[24] Such immune escape variants were found to be genetically stable when processed in tissue culture or retransplanted in animals. An immunochemical analysis of class I MHC antigen expression on the cells revealed that these were neither qualitively nor quantitatively changed when compared to the parental immunosensitive lines. This suggested that immunoselection was directed against the TAA and not against the H-2K restricting molecule.[25] We have recently subjected the immunoresistant variants to 5-azacytidine treatment and cloning and tested their sensitivity to lysis by TAA specific CTL's.[26] Results are shown in Table 1. In about 50% of the subclones we observed reappearance of sensitivity to lysis indicating re-expression of the ESb-specific TAA.

We like to interpret these findings by suggesting that the immunoresistant variants are not real mutants but rather gene regulatory variants. This could explain (1) the high frequency of appearance of the variants during metastasis,[24] (2) the relative stability of the variant phenotype, and (3) the reversibility by using DNA demethylating drugs like 5-azacytidine. This interpretation is illustrated by the model shown in Figure 1.

Regarding the mechanism of generation of tum⁻ variants by alkylating mutagens or 5-azacytidine many questions remain to be answered. The experiments with immunoresistant variants have shown that tumor antigens which were below a threshold of detection by specific T-killer cells can become expressed on such variants in a way

Table 1
RE-EXPRESSION OF TUMOR ANTIGENS ON ESb IMMUNE ESCAPE
VARIANTS AFTER TREATMENT WITH 5-AZACYTIDINE OR MNNG

Tumor line				%[51]Cr release by anti-ESb-CTL[a]	Cold target competition capacity (TAA)[b]
ESb	289		Original line	43.0	+
	775		Immune escape variant	5.0	−
	828		Immune escape varient	3.5	−
			Subclone		
ESb	775-Aza	14		76.5	+
	775-MNNG	1		51.0	+
		5		39.0	+
		7		57.5	+
		8		92.7	+
		11		71.0	+
	828-Aza	9		1.5	−
		21		37.5	+
		24		1.7	−

[a]   DBA/2 anti ESb IL-2 dependent CTL line p76L, effector to target ratio 2:1, 4h cytotoxicity test.
[b]   Cold target competition assay using anti-ESb CTL and ^{51}Cr-labeled ESb 289 target cells. Treated or untreated tumor cell populations were tested to compete with ^{51}Cr-labeled TAA[+] target cells at a ratio of ^{51}Cr target to competitor target of 1:50.

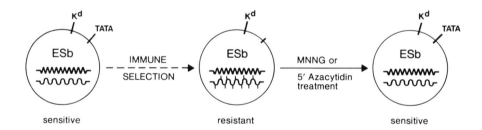

FIGURE 1.   Gene regulatory model for generation of immune escape variants as analyzed in the ESb tumor system. ESb tumor cells are sensitive to lysis by syngeneic CTL which recognize the tumor antigen TATA in association with a K[d] molecule. Upon metastasis from a s.c. inoculation site to the spleen, variants are generated at high frequency which are selectively resistant to tumor specific CTL lysis. K[d] expression is not altered. The model suggest that in these variants the expression of the TATA is down-regulated possibly by DNA methylation. Treatment with DNA demethylating agents leads to re-expression of the TATA and of sensitivity to lysis by tumor specific CTL.

easily detectable by T-killer cells. This may be an example of an induced amplification of expression of already existing determinants.

In addition to such amplified determinants, tum⁻ variants may express new antigenic determinants.[27] This was confirmed recently by us with the parental tumor line Eb and various clones generated by treatment with the drug MNNG (*N*-methyl-*N′*-nitro-*N*-nitrosoguanidine).[28] There were 6 of 18 clones found to be strongly reduced in tumor-igenicity (tum⁻ phenotype). Mice in which such clones had regressed were able to generate tumor specific CTL in vitro. Limiting dilution analysis indicated that three out of four MNNG clones analyzed in detail displayed new antigenic determinants that were detected by CTLP at the clonal level. These new antigens could clearly contribute to the altered immunogenicity. Furthermore, we could provide biochemical evidence for altered cell surface antigens on tum⁻ variants. Membrane proteins of MNNG clones and original Eb cells were compared biochemically after metabolic labeling with ³⁵Smethionine, Triton X 114 solubilization and electrophoretic separation. Two D-gel maps revealed a general quantitative decrease in the expression of membrane proteins in MNNG clones. In addition, several new proteins were found to be expressed. Interestingly, two membrane proteins of 21 and 38 kdaltons were found to be greatly increased in all MNNG clones while they were only weakly expressed in the original Eb cells.[28]

Thus, this analysis revealed multiple cell surface changes in tum⁻ variants including gains and losses of structures and indicated that the effects of mutagens on tumor cells are more complex than so far expected. The amplified cell surface proteins detected could possibly play a role in the altered immunogenicity of the cells. Future experiments will be aimed at a further characterization of cell surface proteins on tum⁻ variants, including studies of transcriptional control of the genes coding for these proteins and on their role in the immunogenicity of the cells. We hope that such a study will help to answer some of the questions relating to the molecular mechanism of generation of tum⁻ variants.

What about the practical applicability of tum⁻ immunogenic tumor variants? Will they help to eradicate micrometastases or minimal residual disease? Can such variants be applied to the treatment of human cancer? Unfortunately, such questions cannot be answered at present but efforts are being made in different laboratories towards their solution.

V. MODULATIONS OF TUMOR CELL IMMUNOGENICITY BY VIRAL XENOGENIZATION

Many efforts have been undertaken in the past to modify tumor cell surfaces to create additional antigenic determinants by chemical modification, enzyme treatment, somatic cell hybridization, or virus infection.[2]

Modification of tumor cells with viruses could be shown to enhance the immunogenicity of several experimental tumors by making them appear "foreign" to the host. Such virus xenogenized tumor cells have been successfully applied for immunotherapy of relatively slow growing experimental tumors[29] and even in man clinical responses were seen in patients bearing melanomas[30] and ovarian carcinomas.[31]

We have tested whether a similar approach could also be successfully applied to fast growing and highly metastatic tumor cells such as the mouse lymphoma ESb. We investigated whether virus modified ESb cells would show increased immunogenicity and could be used for postoperative immunotherapy in animals bearing micrometastases. No curative chemo- or immunotherapy existed so far for this tumor which metastasizes to the liver, lung, spleen, and many other sites.[32] The tumor was xenogenized by infection with an avirulent strain of Newcastle Disease Virus (NDV).

Animals immunized with irradiated virus-infected cells showed increased immunity when compared with animals immunized with irradiated tumor cells alone. The increase of immunogenicity was detected in immunization-protection assays and was confirmed by analyzing the frequency of tumor specific CTLP by limiting dilution analysis (Figure 2). The frequency of tumor specific CTLP could be increased from 1 in 15.300 (ESb immune animals) to 1 in 6.500 (ESb NDV immune animals). The increased CTLP frequency could be due to: (1) activation of CTLP with low affinity for the tumor antigen; (2) activation of helper T-cells leading to extension of CTLP, or (3) to activation via interferon. At the clonal level neither NDV-specific CTL clones nor those recognizing new antigenic determinants could be observed. The cytolytic cells remained highly specific for the tumor antigen of the ESb cells because the parental line Eb from which ESb is a spontaneous variant was not lysed.

When testing the tumor specific CTL response in bulk cultures we again observed an

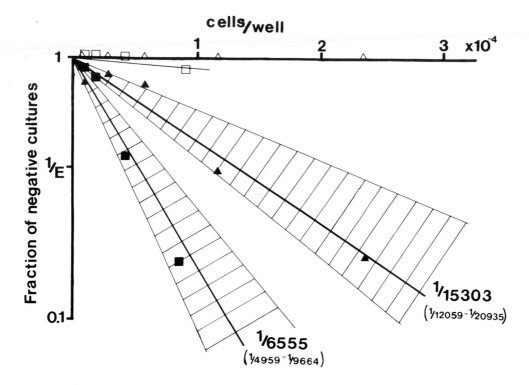

FIGURE 2.   Determination of tumor specific CTLP frequencies by limiting dilution analysis in syngeneic animals immunized against ESb (▲ △) or ESb-NDV (■ □). Spleen cells were removed 9 days after tumor cell inoculation (5×10^4 life cells intrapinna) and graded numbers cultured for 7 days in microtiter plates in the presence of filler cells, IL-2 containing supernatant and mitomycin C treated ESb stimulator cells. Cytotoxic activity of split cultures was determined in a 4 hr ^{51}Cr release assay using as target cells either ESb (▲ ■) or EB (△ □) tumor cells. The figure shows the increase of tumor specific CTLP upon immunization with ESb-NDV as compared to ESb.

increased response (Figure 3). The highest cytotoxicity was seen when NDV infected ESb cells were used both for priming in vivo and for restimulation in vitro. If they were used only once, the response was still better than that obtained with tumor cells without NDV.

Next we investigated the immunotherapeutic capacity of NDV infected ESb tumor cells. The results from two experiments are summarized in Table 2. All animals were inoculated with 5×10^4 ESb cells intradermally. The primary tumor was surgically removed after 10 days when it had reached a size of 5 to 8 mm in diameter. The removal of the primary tumor alone had no or only little curative effect since most of the animals died of disseminated visceral metastases (Table 2, group 2). In contrast, when postoperative immunotherapy was performed with NDV xenogenized autologous tumor cells (group 4), about 50% of the animals survived. Optimal immunotherapy conditions depended on the time of surgery as well as on the concentrations of NDV and tumor cells. In comparison, postoperative immunization with irradiated autologous tumor cells alone (group 3) was ineffective.[34]

Further experiments revealed that animals which had survived due to ESb-NDV therapy had developed long lasting tumor specific systemic immunity.[35] There was no curative effect of this type of therapy in T-cell deficient nude mice suggesting that the effectivity of this approach depended on the presence of T-cells. This does, however, not exclude other types of effector mechanisms such as NK cells or activated macrophages. Such cells might become activated via interferon and could thus contribute to

vitro and in vivo effect of NDV-modification on ESb-specific CTL in syngeneic DBA/2 mice

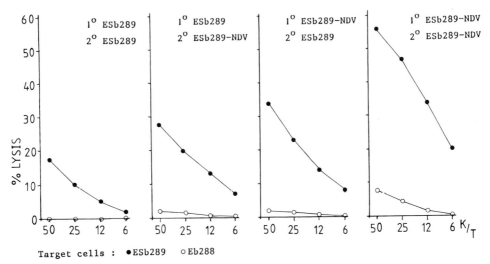

Target cells : •ESb289   ◦Eb288

FIGURE 3.   Increased tumor specific CTL response to NDV modified ESb tumor cells analyzed in bulk cultures. Animals were primed in vivo (1°) as described in Figure 2. Their immune spleen cells were restimulated in vitro (2°) with the indicated stimulator cells for 5 days. Cytotoxic activity was determined in a 4 hr ^{51}Cr release assay.

Table 2

ANTIMETASTATIC THERAPY BY POSTOPERATIVE
IMMUNIZATION WITH VIRUS MODIFIED TUMOR CELLS

				Survivors	
Group	Day 0	Day 10	Therapy	Experiment 1	Experiment 2
1	ESb i.d			0/8	0/8
2	ESb i.d	Surgery		n.d.	2/10
3	ESb i.d	Surgery	ESb 289	0/8	n.d.
4	ESb i.d	Surgery	ESb 289-NDV	4/8	6/9

Note: 5×10^4 tumor cells were inoculated intradermally into the right flank. Animals were operated on day 10 and subsequently treated with 2.5×10^7 irradiated (10,000 rad) ESb 289 cells alone or together with 160 H.U. of NDV s.c. and i.m. Experiments were terminated at day 60 after primary tumor transplant. Data of two experiments are shown.

the effectiveness of this type of therapy. Thus, in this system both natural and specific immune effector mechanisms may contribute to an effective defense against micrometastases. Details of the underlying mechanism of this type of antimetastatic immunotherapy require further elucidation.

We have reviewed several approaches to increase tumor cell immunogenicity and antitumor T-cell reactivity. In contrast to unspecific immune stimulation, the activation of specific T-cell reactivity can lead to long lasting antitumor immunity. In several instances immunization with modified tumor cells led to induction of tumor immunity against the original nonmodified tumor cells. The approaches were also effective with high metastatic tumor lines. For this reason it is hoped that such modified tumor cells could become useful reagents for tumor immunotherapy purposes, especially in situations where the tumor burden is low. Future efforts should be directed towards testing the effectiveness of immunogenic modified tumor variants in combination with surgery or chemotherapy for treatment of micrometastases.

REFERENCES

1. Heppner, G. H. and Miller, B. E., Tumor heterogeneity: biological implications and therapeutic consequences, *Cancer Met. Rev.*, 2, 5, 1983.
2. Schirrmacher, V., Cancer Metastasis: experimental approaches, theoretical concepts, and impacts for treatment strategies, *Adv. Cancer Res.*, 43, 1, 1985.
3. North, R. J., The murine antitumor immune response and its therapeutic manipulation, *Adv. Immunol.*, 35, 89, 1984.
4. Gorelik, E., Concomitant tumor immunity and the resistance to a second tumor challenge, *Adv. Cancer Res.*, 39, 71, 1983.
5. Greenberg, P. D., Kern, D. E., and Cheever, M. A., Therapy of disseminated murine leukemia with cyclophosphamide and immune Lyt 1⁺, 2⁻ T cells, *J. Exp. Med.*, 161, 1122, 1985.
6. Kedar, E. and Weiss, D. W., The in vitro generation of effector lymphyocytes and their employment in tumor immunotherapy, *Adv. Cancer Res.*, 38, 171, 1983.
7. Hewitt, H. B., Animal tumor models for tumor immunology, *J. Biol. Response Modif.*, 1, 107, 1982.
8. Herberman, R. B., Animal tumor models and their relevance to human tumor immunology, *J. Biol. Response Modif.*, 2, 39, 1983.
9. Forni, G. and Santoni, A., Point of view. Immunogenicity of "nonimmunogenic" tumors, *J. Biol. Response Modif.*, 3, 128, 1984.
10. Forni, G., Varesio, L., Giovarelli, M., and Cavallo, D., Dynamic state of spontaneous immune reactivity towards a mammary adenocarcinoma, in *Tumor Antigens and Their Specific Immune Response,* Spreafico, F. and Arnon, R., Eds., Academic Press, New York, 1979, 167.
11. Zoller, M., Evaluation of in vivo and in vitro effectivity of immune defense against a spontaneously arising nonlymphoid rat tumor. II. T cell response after induction of immunogenicity, *Cancer Immunol. Immunother.*, 19, 189, 1985.
12. Lake, P. and Mitchison, N., Regulatory mechanisms in the immune response to cell surface antigens, *Symp. Q. Biol.*, 41, 589, 1976.
13. Rajewsky, K., Schirrmacher, V., Nase, S., and Jerne, N. K., The requirement of more than one antigenic determinant for immunogenicity, *J. Exp. Med.*, 129, 1131, 1969.
14. Zinkernagel, R. M. and Doherty, P. C., MHC-restricted cytotoxic T cells: studies on the biological role of polymorphic major transplantation antigens determining T-cell restriction-specificity, function, and responsiveness, *Adv. Immunol.*, 27, 51, 1979.
15. Schmidt, W., Atfield, G., and Festenstein, H., Loss of H-2Kᵏ gene product(s) from an AKR spontaneous leukaemia, *Immunogenetics*, 8, 311, 1979.
16. Doyle, A., Martin, W. J., Funa, K., Gazdar, A., Carney, D., Martin, S. E., Linnoila, I., Cuttitta, F., Mulshine, J., Bunn, P., and Minna, J., Markedly decreased expression of class I histocompatibility antigens, protein and mRNA in human small-cell lung cancer, *J. Exp. Med.*, 161, 1135, 1985.
17. Hui, K., Grosveld, F., and Festenstein, H., Rejection of transplantable AKR leukaemia cells following MHC DNA-mediated cell transformation, *Nature (London)*, 311, 750, 1984.
18. Wallich, R., Bulbuc, N., Hammerling, G. J., Katzav, S., Segal, S., and Feldman, M., Abrogation of metastatic properties of tumour cells by de novo expression of H-2 K antigens following H-2 gene transfection, *Nature (London)*, 315, 315, 1985.
19. Katzav, S., Segal, S., and Feldman, M., Immuno-selection in vivo of H-2D phenotypic variants from a metastatic clone of sarcoma cells results in cell lines of altered metastatic competence, *Int. J. Cancer*, 33, 407, 1984.
20. Boon, T., Antigenic tumor cell variants obtained with mutagens, *Adv. Cancer Res.*, 39, 121, 1983.
21. Van Pel, A., Vessiere, F., and Boon, T., Protection against two spontaneous mouse leukemias conferred by immunogenic variants obtained by mutagenesis, *J. Exp. Med.*, 157, 1992, 1983.
22. Frost, P., Liteplo, R. G., Donaghue, T. P., and Kerbel, R. S., Selection of strongly immunogenic "tum"-variants from tumors at high frequency using 5-azacytidine, *J. Exp. Med.*, 159, 1491, 1984.
23. Schirrmacher, V., Shantz, G., Clauer, K., Komitowski, D., Zimmermann, H.-P., and Lohmann-Matthes, M. L., Tumor metastases and cell-mediated immunity in a model system in DBA/2 mice. I. Tumor invasiveness in vitro and metastases formation in vivo, *Int. J. Cancer*, 23, 233, 1979.
24. Bosslet, K. and Schirrmacher, V., High-frequency generation of new immunoresistant tumor variants during metastasis of a cloned murine tumor line (ESb), *Int. J. Cancer*, 29, 195, 1982.

25. Altevogt, P., Leidig, S., and Heckl-Oestreicher, B., Resistance of metastatic tumor variants to tumor-specific cytotoxic T-lymphocytes not due to defects in expression of restricting major histocompatibility complex molecules in murine cells, *Cancer Res.*, 44, 5305, 1984.

26. Altevogt, P., von Hoegen, P., and Schirrmacher, V., Treatment of immune-escape tumor variants by 5-Azacytidine or MNNG leads to re-expression of susceptibility to lysis by tumor specific CTL, *Int. J. Cancer*, in press, 1986.

27. Maryanski, J. L. and Boon, T., Immunogenic variants obtained by mutagenesis of mouse mastocytoma P815. IV. Analysis of variant-specific antigens by selection of antigen-loss variants with cytolytic T cell clones, *Eur. J. Immunol.*, 12, 406, 1982.

28. Altevogt, P., von Hoegen, P., Leidig, S., and Schirrmacher, V., Effects of mutagens on the immunogenicity of tumor cells: immunological and biochemical evidence for altered cell surface antigens, *Cancer Res.*, 45, 4270, 1985.

29. Kobayashi, H., Viral xenogenization of intact tumor cells, *Adv. Cancer Res.*, 30, 279, 1979.

30. Wallack, M. K., Meyer, M., Bourgoin, A., Dore, J. F., Leftheriotis, E., Carcagne, J., and Koprowski, H., A preliminary trial of vaccinia oncolysates in the treatment of recurrent melanoma with serologic responses to the treatment, *J. Biol. Response Modif.*, 2, 586, 1983.

31. Lotzova, E., Savary, C. A., Freedman, R. S., and Bowen, J. M., Natural killer cell cytotoxic potential of patients with ovarian carcinoma and its modulation with virus-modified tumor cell extract, *Cancer Immunol. Immunother.*, 17, 124, 1984.

32. Schirrmacher, V., Fogel, M., Russmann, E., Bosslet, K., Altevogt, P., and Beck, L., Antigenic variation in cancer metastasis. Immune escape versus immune control, *Cancer Met. Rev.*, 1, 241, 1982.

33. Karre, K. and Kiessling, R., Personal communication.

34. Heicappell, R., Schirrmacher, V., von Hoegen, P., Ahlert, T., and Appelhans, B., Prevention of metastatic spread by postoperative immunotherapy with virally modified autologous tumor cells. I. Parameters for optimal therapeutic effects, *Int. J. Cancer*, 37, 569, 1986.

35. Shirrmacher, U., Ahlert, T., Heicappel, R., Appelhans, B., and von Hoegen, P., Successful application of nononcogenic viruses for antimetastatic cancer immunotherapy, *Cancer Rev.*, 5, in press, 1986.

Chapter 8

REVIEW OF EVIDENCE FOR ROLE OF NK CELLS IN IMMUNOPRO-PHYLAXIS OF METASTASIS

Nabil Hanna

TABLE OF CONTENTS

I. INTRODUCTION

The development of a metastatic lesion represents the result of a cascade of complex interactions between tumor cells and host defense mechanisms. Both tumor cell properties and host factors influence hematogenous and lymphatic dissemination of malignant neoplasms.[1,2] Considering the complex nature of the metastatic process and the multiple effector mechanisms, immune and nonimmune, involved in host resistance against neoplasia it is not unlikely that certain effector mechanisms may prove effective in limiting the growth and/or spread of tumor cells at different compartments and stages of the metastatic process. For example, natural defense mechanisms may prove effective in destroying circulating tumor cells while exhibiting only a limited effect against extravascular tumor growth. Indeed most tumor cells that enter the circulation are rapidly destroyed and only few survive and succeed to extravasate into the organ parenchyma where they proliferate and develop into metastatic foci.[3-5] Thus, in the context of tumor metastasis one should define the inhibition of tumor cell entry into blood vessels or lymphatic system as well as the destruction of circulating tumor cells before their extravasation into the parenchyma of distant organs as prophylaxis or prevention of tumor metastasis. In contrast, reduction of tumor burden or irradication of established vascularized metastatic growth should be considered and referred to as therapy of tumor metastasis. These are operationally important as different protocols utilizing biologic response modifiers (BRM) which activate different effector mechanisms may be applied for prevention or therapy of tumor metastasis during different stages of the disease. The elucidation of host defense mechanisms that control cancer metastasis is essential for the design of selective antimetastatic therapy as well as for defining the regulatory mechanisms in normal and disease states that influence the activation or suppression of host defenses against metastatic spread of malignant neoplasms.

In this overview the discussion will be focused on the role of NK cells in the inhibition of hematogenous and lymphatic tumor metastasis; their potential role in prevention and therapy of metastasis; the regulatory mechanisms that control NK cell activity in normal and tumor-bearing hosts and on the emergence of NK cell resistance during tumor progression and how it affects tumor metastatic behavior and NK cell-mediated therapy in vivo.

In studying the possible role of NK cells in host defenses against tumor metastasis, most investigators utilized transplantable tumor systems in hosts that exhibit low or high NK cell-mediated cytotoxicity. Also, the ability to selectively activate or deplete NK cells in vivo[5,6] and to conduct adoptive transfer experiments with lymphoid cells or cell lines enriched for NK cell activity[7,8] provided invaluable model systems for evaluating the potential role of NK cells in resistance against tumor growth and metastasis. Among the findings that facilitated the design of experiments which provided most of the evidence for the antimetastatic activity of NK cells are

1. The definition of the critical steps in the metastatic process, their kinetics and sensitivity to selective manipulation of host defenses.[1,2]
2. The discovery of a rapid clearance assay which measures NK cell-mediated destruction of radiolabeled circulating tumor cells in vivo with minimal involvement of macrophages.[5,9]
3. The finding that NK cell activity is dependent upon age, environmental, and genetic factors of the host.[10-12]
4. The in vivo sensitivity of NK cells to hormone and drug treatments (estrogen and cyclophosphamide).[5,13]

5. The presence of antigenic markers (NK-1 and asialo-GM1) which provided reagents for the selective depletion or enrichment of NK effector cells.[14,15]
6. The establishment of cell lines in vitro with NK-like activity and their use for in vivo transfusion studies.[8]
7. The elucidation of the cellular and humoral mechanisms that regulate NK cell activity in vitro and in vivo.
8. The successful selection of tumor cell lines and clones that exhibit high resistance to NK cell-mediated lysis in vitro and high malignant potential in vivo.[16]

Using these model systems, a close correlation between the levels of NK cell activity in the host and the inhibition of metastatic spread of malignant NK-sensitive tumor cells was demonstrated. This finding was further supported by studies in which the metastatic behavior of NK-sensitive and NK-resistant tumor cells was evaluated in hosts that exhibited high or low NK cell levels and by adoptive transfer experiments which provided more direct evidence for the antimetastatic activity of NK cells or NK cell lines in NK-depleted hosts.

II. ENHANCED TUMOR CELL SURVIVAL AND METASTASIS IN MICE WITH LOW LEVELS OF NK CELL-MEDIATED CYTOTOXICITY

NK cell-mediated cytotoxicity in vitro against tumor target cells is markedly inhibited by pretreatment of mice with cyclophosphamide,[5,17] 17-β-estradiol,[13,18] or antiasialo-GM1 serum.[15] In models of experimental metastasis, a single dose of Cy given 4 days before i.v. tumor injection enhanced the incidence of pulmonary and extrapulmonary tumor metastasis of malignant tumor cells.[5] Moreover the survival of radiolabeled tumor cells during the first 24 hr after i.v. inoculation was significantly increased in Cy-treated mice as compared to normal controls. That the Cy-induced enhancement of tumor cell survival and metastasis was caused by depletion of host effector immune cells is supported by adoptive transfer of lymphoid cells.[5] The results of these studies have clearly demonstrated that the Cy effect can be reversed by adoptive transfer of spleen cells from normal, but not from Cy-treated, syngeneic mice or allogeneic nude mice. The transferred lymphoid cells were effective only when administered 4 to 24 hr before, but not after, i.v. tumor cell inoculation. This crucial timing coincides with the presence of tumor cells in the circulation and before their extravasation into the organ parenchyma. Cell fractionation studies demonstrated that the cells active in the reconstitution experiments are non-T, non-B, nonmacrophage, Cy-sensitive, endowed with the ability to kill tumor cells within a short period of time (12 to 24 hr), and share the strain specificity, tissue distribution and ontogenic development described for NK cells.[5] Moreover, selective depletion of NK cells by anti-NK-1.2 serum and complement abolished both the in vitro NK cell-mediated cytotoxicity against the relevant metastatic tumor cells and the antimetastatic activity of normal lymphoid cells transferred to Cy-treated recipients.[19] These findings were further supported by the evidence that in vitro cloned NK-like cell lines upon adoptive transfer to Cy-treated mice enhanced the destruction of circulating radiolabeled tumor cells and inhibited the enhanced lung colonization of malignant murine melanoma cells.[8]

Treatment with antiasialo-GM1 serum and complement inhibits NK cell-mediated killing of lymphoma and solid tumor target cells in vitro.[15] Depletion of NK cells in vivo can also be achieved by i.v. injection of antiasialo-GM1 antibodies.[20] Such treatment resulted in a markedly enhanced survival of radiolabeled circulating tumor cells and increased frequency of pulmonary and extrapulmonary tumor metastases.[7,21,22] Moreover the reduced ability of rats treated with antiasialo-GM1 antibodies to destroy circulating tumor cells could be restored to normal levels by reconstitution with lymphoid populations highly enriched with large granular lymphocytes.[7]

The acute and transient inhibition of NK cell activity by Cy or antiasialo-GM1 serum restricts the utility of these models to short-term studies of experimental metastasis. Alternatively, chronic and selective suppression of NK cell-mediated cytotoxicity in vivo required for the study of spontaneous metastasis may be achieved by treatment with the estrogen, 17-β-estradiol.[13,18,23] The selective inhibition of NK cell activity in β-estradiol-treated mice was associated with increased survival of i.v. inoculated radiolabeled tumor cells and enhanced incidence of both spontaneous and experimental metastasis of the solid tumors UV-2237 fibrosarcoma, K-1735 and B16 melanomas.[23] The enhanced metastatic expression of malignant tumors in estrogen-treated mice could be reversed by adoptive transfer of normal spleen cells. The increased susceptibility of estrogen-treated mice to spontaneous metastasis could not be attributed to enhanced growth rate of the local primary tumors, since the time of appearance of palpable tumors and their growth rate were comparable in β-estradiol-treated and control mice.

Further support of the antimetastatic activity of NK cells was provided by studies using beige mice and 3-week-old mice that naturally exhibit low levels of NK cell-mediated cytotoxicity.[5,24] Several studies have demonstrated that the incidence of experimental and spontaneous metastasis of NK-sensitive B16 melanoma cell line in beige mice was markedly higher than that detected in heterozygous controls.[25] The enhanced pulmonary metastasis correlated with the reduced elimination of radiolabeled tumor cells inoculated i.v. into beige mice, which could be reconstituted to normal levels by adoptive transfer of spleen cells from C57Bl/6 mice. Similar enhancement in the survival of blood borne tumor cells and an increase in the frequency of experimental pulmonary metastasis were observed in young 3-week-old mice that exhibit low levels of NK cell-mediated cytotoxicity in vitro against lymphoma and solid tumor target cells.[5]

Collectively, the evidence presented thus far clearly indicates that the expression of metastatic potential of malignant tumors in vivo is inversely correlated with the levels of host NK cell-mediated cytotoxicity as measured in vitro.

III. ROLE OF NK CELLS IN RESISTANCE OF ATHYMIC NUDE MICE TO TUMOR METASTASIS

Progressive growth of allogeneic and xenogeneic malignant tumors transplanted into nude mice is limited, in most cases, to the site of injection; whereas, metastasis to distant organs is a rare event.[26,27] Local invasiveness and higher incidence of metastasis were observed when newborn[28] or immunosuppressed[29] nude mice were used, suggesting that T-cell independent host defense mechanisms may be responsible for the resistance of nude mice to hematogenous tumor metastasis. The inverse correlation between NK cell levels and incidence of tumor metastasis observed in immuncompetent mice prompted studies of the possible role of NK cells present at high levels in nude mice in the resistance of such recipients to tumor metastasis. Therefore, the levels of NK cell activity and the incidence of experimental and spontaneous metastasis were examined in young 3-week-old nude mice and in adult mice treated with Cy, β-estradiol and antiasialo-GM1.[22,30,31] Low NK cell activity against lymphoma and solid tumor target cells was observed in 3-week-old mice as well as in mice treated with estrogen, Cy, or antiasialo-GM1. Treatment of young nude mice with interferon inducers or bacterial adjuvants boosted their NK cell activity to levels observed in adult mice. These animal models were used to evaluate whether nude mice with low NK cell levels support the growth and dissemination of allogeneic and xenogeneic malignant neoplasms. The i.v. injection of allogeneic murine melanomas and fibrosarcomas and rat adenocarcinomas into young nude mice or mice treated with Cy, antiasialo-GM1, or β-estradiol resulted in enhanced survival of circulating tumor cells and the formation of a large number of lung tumor colonies. In contrast, very few pulmonary tumor metastases developed in untreated adult nude mice injected with equivalent numbers of same tumors. Moreover, activation of NK cells by BRM administered before tumor cell inoculation inhibited the formation of pulmonary metastasis in young nude mice. Chronic depletion of NK cells by β-estradiol or multiple injections of antiasialo-GM1 supported spontaneous metastasis of allogeneic melanoma cells inplanted subcutaneously. Furthermore, the validity of this in vivo model for ascertaining the metastatic potential of tumors is supported by the following observations:

1. The quantitative differences in metastasis formation among tumor cell lines observed in syngeneic hosts were maintained in young nude mice.
2. All metastatic tumors, irrespective of immunogenicity, produced lung colonies in 3-week-old nude mice, whereas nonmetastatic benign tumors did not.
3. Tumor cell lines established from lung metastatic nodules from 3-week-old nude mice injected with allogeneic or xenogeneic (rat) tumors were highly metastatic when reinjected into either young nude mice or syngeneic hosts.[32]

These findings demonstrate that the high metastatic potential of tumor cells isolated from lung metastases is the result of selection rather than adaptation to growth in the nude mouse. Similar studies were carried out using the human melanoma cell line, A-375, where cell lines established from nude mouse lung tumor nodules were more metastatic than the parent line following both i.v. and s.c. injection.[33] Also, Sordat and colleagues[34] have successfully established highly metastasizing sublines from isolated lung metastasis of nude mice injected with a human melanoma cell line. However, further studies with other human cell lines suggested that NK cells may constitute only one factor among several that influence the growth and metastasis of human tumors in athymic nude mice.[35] Overall, these findings support the use of nude mice that exhibit low NK-cell mediated cytotoxicity to ascertain the metastatic potential of human neoplasms and to select for metastatic subpopulations that preexist within the heterogeneous primary tumors.

IV. NK CELL RESISTANCE AND EXPRESSION OF TUMOR MALIGNANCY

Primary tumors are heterogeneous and consist of cell subpopulations that differ in their metastatic potential, antigenic phenotype, and resistance to cytotoxic drugs and immune-mediated mechanisms including NK cell-mediated killing.[2,16,37] Therefore, during the metastatic process host effector mechanisms including NK cells may exert selective pressure on metastasizing tumor cells resulting in the emergence of resistant highly metastatic tumor cell populations. Gorelik and colleagues[37] demonstrated that 3LL carcinoma cells isolated from a spontaneous metastasis were more resistant to killing by NK cells in vitro than cells isolated from the primary tumor. This is by no means without exceptions since many highly metastatic variant cells isolated from pulmonary metastasis of several tumors were as sensitive to NK cell-mediated killing as the parent cell lines.[16] Thus, metastasis is not necessarily the progeny of NK-resistant tumor cells, however, selection for NK-resistant cells may contribute to the expression of the metastatic potential of malignant tumor cells. Considering the many factors involved in the in vivo selection of metastatic tumor cells, an in vitro selection of NK cell resistant tumor cells that may express high metastatic potential in vivo was carried out using the NK-cell-sensitive, poorly metastatic UV-2237 fibrosarcoma.[16] This tumor, however, expresses high metastatic potential when injected into recipients that exhibit low NK cell activity (3-week-old or Cy-treated adult syngeneic mice). The selection of NK-resistant tumor cells was carried out by repeated incubations of the parent UV-2237 cell line with NK cell-enriched spleen cells in vitro. After five successive incubations, the surviving tumor cells (designated NK-5) exhibited a marked resistance to NK cell-mediated lysis in vitro. Following i.v. injection into adult syngeneic mice, the NK-5 cells exhibited an increased survival rate in the pulmonary capillary bed and produced more lung colonies than the NK-sensitive parent tumor cells. Also the NK-5 cells readily metastasized in adult nude mice, known to exhibit high NK cell activity and increased resistance to tumor metastasis. Further characterization of the NK-5 cells indicated that they did not differ from the NK sensitive UV-2237 parent cells in their sensitivity to killing by allogeneic and syngeneic immune T-cells or by activated macrophages. However, they did differ from the parent cells by their inability to bind to NK effector cells in vitro, a property which may be responsible for the selective resistance to NK cell-mediated killing.[58]

Resistance to NK cell-mediated cytotoxicity may also develop during in vivo growth of tumor cells[38,39] which is lost after 2 to 3 weeks of culture in vitro. Following i.v. injection, we observed that the in vivo grown NK-resistant tumor cells survived better in the lung vascular bed and expressed higher metastatic potential in adult syngeneic hosts than the NK sensitive cell line maintained in tissue culture.[25,38] However, no differences in tumor cell survival and lung colonization potential could be observed between the NK-resistant and NK-sensitive counterparts following injection into 3-week-old syngeneic recipients that exhibit low NK cell-mediated activity. Considering that NK resistance may develop as a result of adaptation during in vivo growth of tumor cells or selection during the metastatic process, the therapeutic utility of NK cell activation by BRM should be assessed using in vivo grown NK resistant tumor cells.

V. INHIBITION OF TUMOR METASTASIS BY BRM-MEDIATED ACTIVATION OF NK CELLS

Activation of NK cells may be achieved by interferon, interferon-inducers, bacterial aduvants, and IL-2.[40] Previous studies have demonstrated that administration of NK cell stimuli 1 to 3 days before i.v. tumor cell inoculation markedly reduced the survival of circulating tumor cells and inhibited the development of lung tumor colonies.[5] The antimetastatic effect was most significant when BRM were injected before, but not after, tumor cell inoculation. This is in agreement with previous findings indicating that NK cells are most effective against circulating tumor cells. Although most BRM activate both NK cells and macrophages, albeit with different kinetics, BRM-mediated inhibition of lung colonization and destruction of circulating tumor cells coincided with the kinetics of NK cell, and not macrophage, activation.[6] Also, selective activation of NK cells by certain BRM is sufficient for prevention of experimental tumor metastasis.[6] Moreover, pretreatment of mice with Cy- or β-estradiol abrogates the antimetastatic effect of BRM[5,23] which can be regained by reconstitution with lymphoid populations enriched for NK cells.

More recently evidence was provided for the involvement of NK cells in the antimetastatic effect of anticoagulant drugs.[41] Depletion of NK cells by treatment with antisialo-GM1 antibodies markedly reduced the antimetastatic activity of heparin and prostacylcin. Also, combined treatment with NK stimulants and anticoagulants produced a synergistic effect in enhancement of destruction of circulating tumor cells and inhibition of experimental tumor metastasis.

These findings bear relevance to previous clinical studies in which anticoagulants were used to prevent metastatic spread during surgical removal of the primary tumors.[42] Although at the time of diagnosis, malignant cells may have already metastasized, secondary spread of tumor cells may take place during surgical manipulation of the primary tumor. Thus, monitoring the levels of NK cell activity and applying combined NK cell activation and anticoagulant therapies may prove essential for an effective prevention of secondary metastasis. This becomes more crucial in face of the suppressive effects of surgery and anesthesia on NK cell activity.[43,44]

A common site for spontaneous metastasis from local primary tumor is the lymph nodes. Very early after tumor implantation, tumor cells could be detected in the regional draining lymph nodes.[45] In most cases, however, the early infiltrating cells do not give rise to metastatic foci, and a steady influx of tumor cells from the primary growth is required for metastasis to develop in the lymph nodes. Studies of the role of NK cells in the control of lymph node metastasis showed that treatment with antiasialo-GM1 enhanced both frequency and tumor burden of lymph node metastasis. Alternatively, selective activation of NK cells in lymph nodes containing tumor cells resulted in a marked reduction in tumor burden and metastasis incidence.[58] Similar to results obtained with hematogenous metastasis, BRM treatment was ineffective when initiated at later stages of metastasis development.

The limited efficacy of BRM-activated NK cells in inhibiting the growth of established tumor metastatic foci may be the result of the short duration of NK cell activation observed after a single injection of BRM, the limited ability of activated NK cells to "home" to the metastatic tumor growth during the early stages of its progression and/or the inactivation of NK cells by tumor or host cell products present at high concentrations within the tumor mass. Thus, in addition to studying the homing patterns and anatomical compartmentalization of activated NK cells, the elucidation of the regulatory mechanisms that control NK cell activation is essential for achieving a sustained high level of NK cell activity required for irradiation of established tumor metastases. Moreover, the validity of applying therapeutic protocols developed in normal hosts to tumor-bearing hosts should be critically evaluated.

In an attempt to achieve consistently high levels of activated NK cells, a multiple dosing regimen of BRM was used.[46] From these studies, it became clear that complex cellular interactions regulated BRM-induced NK cell activation. For example, BRM that stimulate NK cell activity may also activate tumoricidal macrophages.[6,46,47] Following the administration of *Corynebacterium parvum,* the early and transient NK cell activation is followed by a prolonged macrophage activation. As is the case with other systems, macrophage activation is associated with the generation of nonspecific suppressor activity mediated by macrophage-like adherent cells which suppress both the inductive and effector phases of NK cell activation.[46,48,49] Thus, following multiple injections of *C. parvum,* a long lasting hyporesponsiveness to reactivation of NK cells was observed.[46] The hyporesponsiveness state corresponded with the kinetics of macrophage activation and suppressor cell induction. These results indicate that multiple injections of certain BRM may not lead to the sustained high levels of NK cell activity required for the control of tumor metastasis. Indeed, BRM were ineffective in preventing lung colonization in hyporesponsive recipients pretreated with *C. parvum.*[46] This reduced antimetastatic activity correlated closely with the emergence of suppressor cells and the inhibition of NK cell activation. The in vivo relevance of this suppressor mechanism was further strengthened by studies in which normal spleen cells failed to restore the suppressed NK cell activity or NK cell-mediated inhibition of tumor metastasis following adoptive transfer into *C. parvum*-pretreated hyporesponsive recipients. Although the mechanisms of suppression are not fully elucidated, previous studies indicated that prostaglandins are involved in macrophage-mediated suppression and treatment with cyclooxygenase inhibitors inhibited the expression of such suppressive mechanisms in several systems.[50,51]

Suppressor mechanisms that inhibit NK cell activity were described also in tumor-bearing hosts.[50] In recent studies we have demonstrated that BRM-induced activation of NK cells in vitro and in vivo is markedly inhibited in tumor-bearing mice. Suppressor adherent cells were detected in animals bearing relatively large (>1.0 cm) tumors (UV-2237 fibrosarcoma). This suppression could be reversed by either removal of the adherent cell population or treatment with indomethacin in vitro. However, at later stages of tumor development the inhibition of NK cell activation could not be attributed to the presence of suppressor cells only and additional mechanisms of NK cell inactivation or depletion were postulated. Studies in vivo have demonstrated that clearance of i.v. injected radiolabeled tumor cells in untreated or BRM-treated tumor-bearing mice was markedly reduced as compared with normal control mice. The reduced clearance of circulating tumor cells correlated closely with the suppression of NK cells in animals bearing large tumors. These findings clearly indicate that monitoring suppressor cells and implementing strategies for modulating their function are essential for the design of effective immune-mediated therapy of cancer metastasis.

Because of the complex cellular interactions involved in the regulation of NK cell activity, the selective activation of NK cells without subsequent activation of suppressor macrophages may prove superior for evaluating the potential of NK cell activation in therapy of established tumor micrometastasis. For example, periodate-oxidized *C. parvum* did not activate tumoricidal macrophages but retained the NK-stimulating capacity of untreated *C. parvum*.[6] The enhanced NK cell-mediated cytotoxicity was manifested in vivo by increased destruction of radiolabeled circulating tumor cells and inhibition of hematogenous and lymph node metastasis. Furthermore, unlike untreated *C. parvum,* the periodate-oxidized bacteria failed to activate suppressor macrophages or to induce hyporesponsiveness to further activation of NK cells and to BRM-mediated inhibition of experimental metastasis.[46]

A critical factor in tumor immunotherapy is the ability to activate effector cells that reside within the tumor mass or, alternatively, to mobilize systemically activated effector mechanisms to the site of metastatic tumor growth. Indeed, investigation of NK cell activity of tumor-associated lymphocytes isolated from human solid tumors revealed low or no detectable cytotoxicity caused primarily by the apparent low frequency of effector NK cells in such lymphoid populations.[52] Thus, elucidation of the organ localization and circulatory patterns of activated NK cells may contribute to the design of effective immunotherapy of extravascular metastatic tumor growth.

Studies of the regulation of lymph node NK cell activation revealed that the tissue distribution and kinetics of NK cell activation or suppression varied according to the type, dose and route of administration of the BRM.[53] Thus, intrafootpad injection of *C. parvum* resulted in activation of NK cells in the regional popliteal lymph nodes, peripheral blood, and spleen; whereas, contralateral and distant lymph nodes were negative. Similarly, i.v., injection of low doses of *C. parvum* activated NK cells in peripheral blood and spleen but not in popliteal lymph nodes. In contrast, treatment with potent interferon inducers such as poly I.C1-C activated NK cells in all compartments tested. These findings strongly suggest that activated NK cells display a restricted circulatory pattern which renders it difficult to predict the levels of activated NK cells at the site of tumor metastasis by monitoring NK cell activity in peripheral blood. As described before, only BRM treatment protocols that activate NK cells in lymph nodes draining the primary tumor growth inhibited the development of lymph node metastasis. In a more recent study it was demonstrated that augmented NK cell activity in the lung and liver observed following BRM treatment correlated with the resistance against the development of tumor metastasis in those organs.[54] Similarly, the depletion of organ-associated NK cells by high doses of antiasialo GM1 resulted in a marked enhancement in the survival of tumor cells lodged in the vascular bed of these organs.[55]

Successful NK cell-mediated immunotherapy of tumor metastasis also depends on the relative sensitivity of tumor cells to NK cell-mediated killing. As discussed above, in vivo grown tumor cells are more resistant to killing by endogenous NK cells in vitro and produce more lung colonies in vivo than their cultured counterparts.[39] However, recent studies have demonstrated that freshly excised human and murine tumor cells, although resistant to killing by unactivated endogenous NK cells, were sensitive to lysis by BRM-activated NK cells in vitro[39,56,57] and their metastases were markedly inhibited by in vivo activation of host NK cells.[39] Similarly, the in vitro selected NK-resistant and highly metastatic murine NK-5 cell line was sensitive in vitro and in vivo, to lysis of BRM-activated, but not endogenous, NK cells. Thus, the emergence of NK cell resistance during the metastatic process should not interfere with the antimetastatic activity of BRM-activated NK cells and therefore should not curtail efforts of applying such protocols to the control of tumor micrometastasis.

In summary, although the therapeutic efficacy of NK cells in the control of established tumor metastasis awaits further proof, their role in the immunoprophylaxis of hematogenous and lymphatic spread of malignant neoplasmas is well established. Moreover, protocols designed to selectively activate NK cells may achieve the sustained activation required for therapy of established micrometastasis.

REFERENCES

1. Fidler, I. J., Gersten, D. M., and Hart, I. R., The biology of cancer invasion and metastasis, *Adv. Cancer Res.*, 28, 149, 1978.
2. Poste, G. and Fidler, I. J., The pathogenesis of cancer metastasis, *Nature (London)*, 283, 139, 1980.
3. Fidler, I. J., Metastasis: quantitative analysis of distribution and fate of tumor emboli labeled with ^{125}I-5liodo-2'deoxyuridine, *J. Natl. Cancer Inst.*, 45, 733, 1970.
4. Liotta, L. A., Kleinerman, J., and Saidel, G. M., Quantitative relationships of intravascular tumor cells, tumor vessels and pulmonary metastasis following tumor implantation, *Cancer Res.*, 34, 997, 1974.
5. Hanna, N. and Fidler, I. J., The role of natural killer cells in the destruction of circulating tumor emboli, *J. Natl. Cancer Inst.*, 65, 801, 1980.
6. Hanna, N., Inhibition of experimental tumor metastasis by selective activation of natural killer cells, *Cancer Res.*, 42, 1337, 1982.
7. Barlozzari, T., Reynolds, C. W., and Herberman, R. B., In vivo role of natural killer cells; involvement of large granular lymphocytes in the clearance of tumor cells in anti-asialo GM1-treated rats, *J. Immunol.*, 131(2), 1024, 1983.
8. Warner, J. and Dennert, G., Effects of a cloned cell line with NK activity on bone marrow transplants, tumour development and metastasis *in vivo*, *Nature (London)*, 300, 31, 1982.
9. Riccardi, C., Puccetti, P., Santoni, A., and Herberman, R. B., Rapid *in vivo* assay of mouse natural killer cell activity, *J. Natl. Cancer Inst.*, 63, 1041, 1979.
10. Herberman, R. B., Ninn, M. E., and Laurin, D. H., Natural cytotoxic reactivity of mouse lymphoid cells against syngeneic and allogeneic tumors. I. Distribution of reactivity and specificity, *Int. J. Cancer*, 16, 216, 1975.
11. Keissling, R., Klein, E., and Wigzell, H., Natural killer cells in the mouse. I. Cytotoxic cells with specificity for mouse Moloney leukemia cells. Specificity and distribution according to genotype, *Eur. J. Immunol.*, 5, 112, 1975.
12. Hanna, N., Davis, T. W., and Fidler, I. J., Environmental and genetic factors determine the level of NK activity of nude mice and affect their suitability as models for experimental metastasis, *Int. J. Cancer*, 30, 371, 1982.
13. Seaman, W. E., Blackman, M. A., Gindhart, T. D., Roubinia, J. R., Loeb, J. M., and Talal, N., β-estradiol reduces natural killer cells in mice, *J. Immunol.*, 121, 2193, 1978.
14. Burton, R. C., Alloantisera selectively reactive with NK cells: characterization and use in defining NK cell classes, in *Natural Cell Mediated Immunity to Tumors*, Herberman, R. B., Ed., Academic Press, New York, 1980, 19.

15. Young, W. W., Hakomori, S. I., Durdik, J. M., and Henney, C. S., Identification of ganglio-N-tetraosylceramide as a new cell surface marker for murine natural killer (NK) cells, *J. Immunol.*, 124, 199, 1980.

16. Hanna, N. and Fidler, I. J., Relationship between metastatic potential and resistance to natural killer cell-mediated cytotoxicity in three murine tumor systems, *J. Natl. Cancer Inst.*, 66, 1183, 1981.

17. Mantovani, A., Luini, W., Peri, G., Vecchi, A., and Spraefico, F., Effect of chemotherapeutic agents on natural cell-mediated cytotoxicity in mice, *J. Natl. Cancer Inst.*, 61, 1255, 1978.

18. Kalland, T. and Fosberg, J. G., Natural killer cell activity and tumor susceptibility in female mice treated neonatally with diethylstilbestrol, *Cancer Res.*, 41, 5134, 1981.

19. Hanna, N. and Burton, R. C., Definitive evidence that natural killer (NK) cells inhibit tumor metastasis *in vivo, J. Immunol.*, 127, 1754, 1981.

20. Kasai, M., Yoneda, T., Habu, S., Maruyama, Y., Okumura, K., and Tokunaga, T., *In vivo* effect of anti-asialo GM1 antibody on natural killer activity, *Nature (London)*, 291, 334, 1981.

21. Gorelik, E., Wiltrout, R., Okumura, K., Habu, S., and Herberman, R. B., Acceleration of metastatic growth in anti-asialo GM1-treated mice, in *NK Cells and Other Natural Effector Cells*, Herberman, R. B., Ed., Academic Press, New York, 1982, 1331.

22. Hanna, N., Natural killer cell-mediated inhibition of tumor metastasis *in vivo, Surv. Synth. Pathol. Res.*, 2, 68, 1983.

23. Hanna, N. and Schneider, M., Enhancement of tumor metastasis and suppression of natural killer cell activity by β-estradiol treatment, *J. Immunol.*, 130, 974, 1980.

24. Roder, J. and Duwe, A., The beige mutation in the mouse selectively impairs natural killer cell function, *Nature (London)*, 278, 451, 1979.

25. Talmadge, J. E., Meyers, K. M., Prieur, D. J., and Starkey, J. R., Role of NK cells in tumor growth and metastasis in beige mice, *Nature (London)*, 284, 622, 1980.

26. Fidler, I. J., Caines, G., and Dolan, Z., Survival of hematogenously disseminated allogeneic tumor cells in athymic nude mice, *Transplantation*, 22, 208, 1976.

27. Povlsen, C. O., Heterotransplantation of human malignant melanomas to the mouse mutant nude, *Acta Pathol. Microbiol. Scand. A*, 84, 9, 1976.

28. Sordat, B., Merenda, C., and Carrel, S., Invasive growth and dissemination of human solid tumors and malignant cell lines grafted subcutaneously to new born nude mice, in *Proc. 2nd Int. Workshop N M*, Nomura, T., Ohsawa, N., Tamaoki, N., and Fujiwara, K., Eds., University of Tokyo Press, Tokyo, 1977, 313.

29. Reid, L. M., Holland, J., Jones, C., Wolf, B., and Sato, G., Some of the variables affecting the success of transplantation of human tumors into the athymic nude mouse, in *Proc. Symp. Use Athymic (Nude) Mice Cancer Res.*, Houchens, D. P. and Ovejera, A. A., Eds., Gustav Fischer Verlag, New York, 1978, 107.

30. Hanna, N. and Fidler, I. J., Expression of metastatic potential of allogeneic and xenogeneic neoplasms in young nude mice, *Cancer Res.*, 41, 438, 1981.

31. Hanna, N., Expression of metastatic potential of tumor cells in young nude mice is correlated with low levels of natural killer cell-mediated cytotoxicity, *Int. J. Cancer*, 26, 675, 1980.

32. Pollack, V. A. and Fidler, I. J., The use of young nude mice to select subpopulations of tumor cells with increased metastatic potential from nonsyngeneic neoplasms, *J. Natl. Cancer Inst.*, 69, 137, 1982.

33. Kozlowski, J. M., Hart, I. R., Fidler, I. J., and Hanna, N., A human melanoma line heterogeneous with respect to metastatic capacity in athymic nude mice, *J. Natl. Cancer Inst.*, 72, 913, 1984.

34. Sordat, B. C. M., Ueyama, Y., and Fogh, J., Metastasis of tumor xenografts in the nude mouse, in *The Nude Mouse in Experimental and Clinical Research*, Fogh, J. and Giovanella, B. C., Eds., Academic Press, New York, 1982, 95.

35. Kozlowski, J. M., Fidler, I. J., Campbell, D., Xu, Z. L., Kaighn, M. E., and Hart, I. R., Metastatic behavior of human cell lines grown in the nude mouse, *Cancer Res.*, 44, 3522, 1984.

36. Fidler, I. J., Tumor heterogeneity and the biology of cancer invasion and metastasis, *Cancer Res.*, 38, 2651, 1978.

37. Gorelick, E., Fogel, M., Feldman, M., and Segal, S., Differences in resistance of metastatic tumor cells and cells from local tumor growth to cytotoxicity of natural killer cells, *J. Natl. Cancer Inst.*, 63, 1397, 1979.

38. Becker, S., Kiessling, R., Lee, N., and Klein, G., Modulation of sensitivity to natural killer cell lysis after *in vitro* explanation of a mouse lymphoma, *J. Natl. Cancer Inst.*, 61, 1495, 1978.

39. Hanna, N., Role of natural killer cells in control of cancer metastasis, *Cancer Met. Rev.*, 1, 45, 1982.

40. Trinchieri, G. and Perussia, B., Human natural killer cells: biologic and pathologic aspects, *Lab. Invest.*, 50, 489, 1984.

41. Gorelik, E., Bere, W. W., and Herberman, R. B., Role of NK cells in the antimetastatic effect of anticoagulant drugs, *Int. J. Cancer*, 33, 87, 1984.

42. Hoover, H. C., Ketcham, A. S., Millar, R. C., and Gralnick, H. R., Osteosarcoma: improved survival with anticoagulation and amputation, *Cancer,* 41, 2475, 1978.
43. Pollock, R. E., Babcock, G. F., Romsdahl, M. M., and Nishioka, K., Surgical stress-mediated suppression of murine natural killer cell cytotoxicity, *Cancer Res.,* 44, 3888, 1984.
44. Shapiro, J., Jersky, J., Katzav, S., Feldman, M., and Segal, S., Anesthetic drugs accelerate the progression of postoperative metastases of mouse tumors, *J. Clin. Invest.,* 68, 678, 1981.
45. Carr, I., Lymphatic metastasis, *Cancer Met. Rev.,* 2, 307, 1983.
46. Hanna, N., Regulation of natural killer cell activation: implementation for the control of tumor metastasis, *Natl. Immun. Cell Growth Regul.,* 3, 22, 1984.
47. Puccetti, P., Santoni, A., Riccardi, C., Holden, H., and Herberman, R. B., Activation of mouse macrophages by pyran copolymer and role in augmentation of natural killer activity, *Int. J. Cancer,* 24, 819, 1979.
48. Lotzova, E., *C. parvum*-mediated suppression of the phenomenon of natural killing and its analysis, in *Natural Cell-Mediated Immunity Against Tumors,* Herberman, R. B., Eds., Academic Press, New York, 1980, 735.
49. Santoni, A., Riccardi, C., Barlozzani, T., and Herberman, R. B., Suppression of activity of mouse natural killer (NK) cells by activated macrophages from mice treated with pyran copolymer, *Int. J. Cancer,* 26, 837, 1980.
50. Brunda, M. J., Herberman, R. B., and Holden, H. T., Inhibition of murine natural killer cell activity by prostaglandins, *J. Immunol.,* 124, 2682, 1980.
51. Brunda, M. J. and Holden, H. T., Prostaglandin-mediated inhibition of murine natural killer cell activity, in *Natural Cell-Mediated Immunity Against Tumors,* Herberman, R. B., Ed., Academic Press, New York, 1980, 721.
52. Introna, M. and Mantovani, A., Natural killer cells in human solid tumors, *Cancer Met. Rev.,* 2, 337, 1983.
53. Hisano, G. and Hanna, N., Murine lymph node natural killer cells: regulatory mechanisms of activation or suppression, *J. Natl. Cancer Inst.,* 69, 665, 1982.
54. Wiltrout, R. H., Mathieson, B. J., Talmadge, J. E., Reynolds, C. W., Zhang, S. R., Herberman, R. B., and Ortaldo, J. R., Augmentation of organ-associated natural killer activity by biological response modifiers. Isolation and characterization of large granular lymphocytes from the liver, *J. Exp. Med.,* 160, 1431, 1984.
55. Wiltrout, R. H., Herberman, R. B., Zhang, S. R., Chirigos, M. A., Ortaldo, J. R., Green, K. M., and Talmadge, J. A., Role of organ-associated NK cells in decreased formation of experimental metastases in lung and liver, *J. Immunol.,* 134, 4267, 1985.
56. Moore, M., Taylor, G. M., and White, W. J., Susceptibility of human leukemias to cell-mediated cytotoxicity by interferon-treated allogeneic lymphocytes, *Cancer Immunol. Immunother.,* 13, 56, 1982.
57. Pattengale, P. K., Gidlung, M., Nilsson, K., Sundstrom, C., Sallstrom, J., Simonsson, B., and Wigzell, H., Lysis of fresh human β-lymphocyte-derived leukemia cells by interferon-activated natural killer (NK) cells, *Int. J. Cancer,* 29, 1, 1982.
58. Hanna, N., Unpublished observations.

Chapter 9

ROLE OF NK CELLS IN PREVENTION AND TREATMENT OF METASTASES BY BIOLOGICAL RESPONSE MODIFIERS

Robert H. Wiltrout, James E. Talmadge, and Ronald B. Herberman

TABLE OF CONTENTS

I. INTRODUCTION

Cancer metastasis is the result of a sequence of events which are dependent on inherent properties of tumor cells and on a series of interactions between tumor cells and their host.[1-3] This process is a continuum that can be artificially divided into five steps:

1. Growth of the primary tumor, followed by invasion of cells from the primary tumor into the surrounding tissue to gain access into blood and/or lymphatic vessels.
2. Release of tumor cell emboli into the circulation.
3. Arrest of emboli in distant organs.
4. Tumor cell invasion (extravasation) into the organ parenchyma followed by proliferation.
5. Growth of vascularized stroma into the new tumor focus.

The entire process may then be repeated to produce secondary metastases.

The outcome of the interaction between the metastatic tumor cell and the host is largely predicated on the tumor cell possessing the necessary biochemical and physical attributes required for completing all aspects of the metastatic process, the so-called metastatic phenotype.[1-3] Since components of the immune system can interact with disseminating tumor cells at several stages of the metastatic cascade, one aspect of the metastatic phenotype is the ability of the disseminating tumor cell to circumvent host immune defenses.

For simplicity, we will consider the process of metastasis to be a progression of tumor dissemination among three anatomical compartments. The first compartment is the organ-site of origin of the primary tumor. Since metastasis often proceeds by hematogenous spread, the second compartment considered will be the vascular system, including the capillaries and venules in the target organs to which the tumor cell(s) may disseminate. The third compartment will be considered to be the parenchyma of the organ tissue in which the metastasis will develop, including the process of extravasation from the vasculature. Inhibition of metastasis formation by the immune system could result from destruction of metastasizing tumor cells in any of these three compartments, whereas immunotherapy of established metastases would be dependent on affecting the target organ which contains established tumor foci. In this chapter we will focus on the role of NK cells in augmented resistance to metastasis formation and/or progression following treatment of the host with BRMs.

NK cells are defined as effector cells which mediate spontaneous cytotoxic activity against various targets without restriction related to the MHC, and which lack the properties of classical macrophages, granulocytes, or CTL.[4] Further it is now possible to isolate highly enriched lymphocyte populations and show that NK activity is closely associated with a subpopulation of lymphocytes, morphologically identified as large granular lymphocytes (LGL), that comprise about 5% of peripheral blood or splenic lymphocytes and 1 to 3% of total mononuclear cells. LGL have been isolated by discontinuous density gradient centrifugation on Percoll from the blood or spleens of humans,[5,6] rats,[7] and mice,[8-10] and they also have been isolated or identified in the small intestine,[11,12] lungs,[3] and liver.[10,14,15] However, the number and percentages of LGL may vary greatly among these anatomical compartments.[16] LGL contain azurophilic cytoplasmic granules, are nonphagocytic, nonadherent cells that lack surface immunoglobulin but contain cell-surface receptors for the Fc portion of IgG. Some cell surface antigens, particularly those detected by monoclonal antibodies, have been found on at least a portion of LGL and these have been very helpful in characterizing the phenotype of NK cells. In mice, about half of the NK cells in the spleen have been shown to express low levels of Thy 1 antigen.[4] The glycolipid asialo GM-1 has also been shown to be a rather selective marker for the majority of NK cells.[17] In rats, most of the LGL have been found to express the OX8 antigen,[18] which is also associated with the cytotoxic/suppressor subset of T-cells. These findings, along with the demonstration of high levels of NK activity in nude[19] or neonatally thymectomized mice[20] or nude rats,[21] are compatible with the hypothesis that NK cells represent a side path way of differentiation from prethymic cells in the T-cell lineage. Alternatively, it is possible that NK cells are derived from an independent lineage of stem cells and simply share some characteristics with, and are regulated by, T-cells.

Consistent with the possibility of a relationship of NK cells to the T-cell lineage, NK cells have been shown to respond to IL-2 and can grow and be maintained in culture. Cell cultures initiated from highly purified LGL retain their morphologic and cytotoxic characteristics.[22] In addition to the ability of IL-2 to promote the proliferation of NK cells, IL-2 has been found to strongly augment the cytotoxic activity of both mouse and human NK cells, IL-2 has been found to strongly augment both mouse and human NK activity.[23] The IL-2 boosting of NK activity appears to result from a direct interaction of the lymphokine with LGL.[23] Recent evidence also indicates that at least some of the tumoricidal activity of lymphokine activated killer (LAK) cells in the human results from stimulation of Leu 11[+], NK-active LGL by IL-2.[24]

Interferon (IFN) also has been shown to potently augment the activity of NK cells. In vivo administration to mice or rats of a variety of IFN-inducers, or of IFN itself, led to rapid boosting of NK activity. Similarly, incubation in vitro of human or rodent lymphoid cells or of purified LGL with IFN induced considerable augmentation of NK activity.[25,26]

The properties of spontaneous cytotoxicity, rapid augmentation of tumoricidal activity by endogenously produced BRMs like IL-2 and IFN, and a proliferative response following stimulation by IL-2, make NK cells attractive candidates for an immunosurveillance role against cancer development or spread. There is considerable evidence that NK cells are important for the prevention of metastases in normal animals, and that the augmentation or depression of NK activity in lymphoid organs and the blood correlates with increased or decreased resistance to metastases, respectively.[27,28] (Also see Chapter 8.) In this chapter, we will review the evidence that NK cells exist in nonlymphoid organs which are often sites for the formation of metastases, that NK activity in these organs can be potently augmented by administration of BRMs, and that this augmentation of organ-associated NK activity contributes to the antimetastatic effects associated with BRM-administration.

II. AUGMENTATION OF NK ACTIVITY IN DIFFERENT ANATOMICAL COMPARTMENTS

Most studies of immune function, including assessment of NK activity, are routinely performed by evaluating activities in three sites: blood, spleen, or peritoneal cavity. While there are substantial logistical and ethical reasons for this limited immune monitoring, it is quite possible that the most important effects of a BRM are not associated with changes in the immune status in these sites. For example, metastases are most frequently located in vital nonlymphoid organs where they may not be sufficiently accessible to treatment with surgery or chemotherapy. Perhaps the strongest rationale for the development of immunotherapeutic treatment protocols is the hope that the immune system can be utilized to control minimal residual disease in inaccessible tumor foci, as an adjunct to conventional forms of cancer treatment. Therefore, it is imperative to determine whether the immunomodulatory effects of BRMs on lymphoid compartments like the spleen are also observed in more therapeutically relevant sites like the lungs and the liver. Such information is critical for the rational design of therapeutic strategies for cancer treatment by BRMs, and for evaluating the effectiveness of such trials.

A. Augmentation of NK Activity in Lymphoid and Nonlymphoid Organs

Numerous synthetic, microbially derived, or host-derived BRMs have been demonstrated to augment to varying degrees the NK activity in lymphoid organs. In general, these BRMs fall into two categories based primarily on the mechanism by which they augment NK activity. The first group of NK-augmenting BRMs augment NK activity largely as a result of IFN production.[23,25,26,29-33] This group consists mostly of viruses, synthetic compounds, and bacterially derived products. The second group of agents may augment NK activity at least partially by IFN-independent mechanisms.[28,30,34] This group includes cytokine/hormone BRMs such as IL-2[23,34-36] and β-endorphin;[37,38] heavy metals;[39] the bacterial BRM OK-432;[40] or antibodies with specificity for H-2, Ia, or Thy-1 antigens.[41]

Additionally, it has been demonstrated that viruses[42-46] and parasites[47] preferentially augment NK activity in localized compartments. Therefore, we designed studies to determine whether BRMs could augment NK activity in major nonlymphoid organs like the lungs and the liver. The intitial studies demonstrated that both the pyran copolymer, maleic anhydride divinyl ether (MVE-2), and a killed preparation of the bacteria, *Propionibacterium acnes (P. acnes),* potently augmented NK activity in the livers of mice.[10] More recently we have also found that poly I:C/L:C,[48] OK-432,[49,50] and human recombinant IL-2[51,52] also augmented hepatic NK activity to a greater extent than that observed in the more commonly examined sites, such as blood and spleen. Further studies in mice have extended these observations to the lungs, where we have also observed an increased augmentation of NK activity over that observed in blood and spleen.[52-54] In the liver the cause of the augmented NK activity is associated with a 10- to 50-fold increase in the total number of isolatable LGL.[10] Similarly Hurme et al.,[55] have recently reported that poly I:C induces an increase in the number of LGLs that are isolatable from the lungs. In our studies the total number of LGL, and the percent of LGL among the total nonparenchymal cells (NPC) in the liver, were found to be dependent on the BRM administered[10,49,50] and the time after BRM administration when cells were isolated. In general, peak numbers of LGL were reached 1 to 4 days after BRM administration and gradually returned to baseline levels thereafter.

Previous observations demonstrated that the repeated administration of IFN during preclinical,[56] clinical trials,[57,58] or of MVE-2 to mice,[59,60] resulted in a hyporesponsiveness to augmentation of NK activity in the blood and/or spleen. This hyporesponsive state was characterized by an inability of repeated administrations of the BRM to augment NK activity to the levels achieved by a single administration. In fact, in some instances the levels of NK activity in the blood and/or spleen were less than those observed in untreated control mice[59,60] or in patients prior to treatment.[57] Further studies indicated that some BRMs, most notably *P. acnes*, were able to induce a transient augmentation of NK activity in the spleen and peritoneal cavity of mice, followed by a hyporesponsiveness to restimulation by the same or another BRM.[61] Subsequently, it has been shown that this hyporesponsiveness to augmentation of blood and splenic NK activity by *P. acnes* was at least partially due to the presence of suppressor cells.[62,63] To determine whether this hyporesponsiveness was systemic or restricted to specific compartments, we examined NK activity in both the routinely monitored sites (blood and spleen) as well as in a nonlymphoid organ compartment (liver) following repeated administration of various BRMs. Repeated administration of MVE-2,[28,57] poly ICLC, or OK-432[52] resulted in sustained high levels of NK activity in the lungs and liver, whereas the IFNs were found to induce systemic NK hyporesponsiveness.[52]

Cumulatively, the evidence indicates that many BRMs are capable of augmenting NK activity in nonlymphoid organs to a greater degree than in the blood and spleen. Some BRMs are capable of maintaining augmented organ-associated NK activity following repeated administration, in contrast to the usual lack of augmented NK activity in the blood or spleen following repeated administration of the same BRMs. These observations indicate that the NK-mediated antimetastatic effects of a BRM may be more pronounced in sites of metastasis formation than those that occur in the blood during the intravascular phase of the metastatic process. The results further suggest that by understanding the ability of different BRMs to augment NK activity in various compartments, it may be possible to select certain BRMs that may induce immune modulation in the desired sites, i.e., in areas of primary tumor growth or metastasis.

B. Mechanisms by Which NK Activity is Augmented in Organs

There are several possible ways in which administration of BRMs may cause an increase in the total NK activity of an organ. The first possibility would be by simply increasing the activation state of the existing NK cells. Second, BRMs could cause an increase in the total number of organ-associated NK cells. This increase could result from BRM-induced differentiation of NK precursors, stimulation of proliferation by NK cells, or by a recruitment and influx of NK cells from other sites. The fact that many BRMs rapidly augment NK activity in vitro[34] is consistent with the expectation that they may also do this in vivo. However, our studies have clearly demonstrated that following administration of MVE-2 or *P. acnes*, there is a rapid increase in the number of LGL which we can isolate from the liver[10,50] and therefore in vivo augmentation of NK activity probably is attributable to an increase in the effector cell population as well as to an increase in activity of pre-existent effector cells.

Stimulation of LGL proliferation also was observed in the studies of Biron et al.[64] Mice infected with lymphocytic choriomeningitis virus (LCMV) were found to have large blast-like cells, which incorporated ³H-thymidine and lysed the NK-susceptible YAC-1 tumor cell line.[64] Further, the generation of these cells following LCMV infection was blocked by γ-irradiation or by hydroxyurea, which arrests cells at the G1/S interphase.[65] In addition, Santoni et al. have recently reported that a variety of BRMs, including *P. acnes*, MVE-2, poly I:C, and IFN augment NK activity, increase the percentage of LGL, and increase the number of lower density LGL in the spleens of mice.[66] An increased proportion of such cells incorporated ³H-thymidine and were shown to be in S phase. Also, recent results demonstrating that IL-2 causes NK cells to proliferate in vitro[22] suggest that BRM-induced lymphokines might also induce NK cell proliferation in vivo. In fact, our studies have demonstrated that some of the LGL isolated from the livers of MVE-2 treated mice are proliferating.[28] Overall, these results indicate that in vivo augmentation of NK activity is at least partially due to a BRM-induced proliferation of NK cells. However, in addition, histological of analyses of the livers of MVE-2 treated mice revealed the presence of a mononuclear infiltrate,[28] while similar studies in athymic rats confirmed the presence of OX-8⁺ NK cells in the infiltrate.[126] We have also demonstrated that purified LGL isolated from peripheral blood localized in significant numbers in livers of rats following i.v. injection.[67] Further, this localization of both purified normal splenic LGL and MVE-2 liver-derived LGL was greater in the livers of BRM-treated mice than it was in normal mice following i.v. injection.[127]

Therefore, the available evidence suggests that the BRM-induced increase in NK activity in the liver is partially due to an increase in LGL which occurs by a combination of proliferation and influx of LGL via the blood. Further, the results suggest that the hyporesponsiveness of NK activity which is induced in blood and spleen by repeated administration of some BRMs,[56-60] may be partially due to a redistribution or diversion of NK cells from those sites.[52]

III. RELATIONSHIP BETWEEN LEVELS OF NK ACTIVITY AND RESISTANCE TO METASTASIS FORMATION

A. Metastatic Potential of NK-Resistant vs. NK-Susceptible Tumors

Highly metastatic cells differ from the parental tumor in a variety of ways, many of which could contribute to the successful formation of a metastasis. Resistance or susceptibility of tumor cells to NK activity may be one of the parameters which influence metastatic potential. This possibility could be tested in several ways. For example, the prediction that NK-susceptible tumors would metastasize less than NK-resistant variants could be evaluated. Similarly, one could determine whether cells which have successfully metastasized would in general be more NK-resistant than the unselected parental primary tumor. In general, the predicted correlations have been observed in a variety of studies.[68-72] These results indicate that selection by the host of tumor sublines resistant to NK activity contributes to, but is not sufficient for, expression of enhanced metastatic potential.

Another approach to investigating the relationship between NK-resistant of tumor cells and their metastatic potential has been to select for tumor cells with enhanced metastatic ability and assess the relative susceptibility of these cells to NK activity. If resistance to NK activity contributes to enhanced metastases, then highly metastatic tumors or their metastases should be more NK-resistant than less metastatic tumors or primary tumors. Several groups have presented evidence to support the conclusion that highly metastatic tumor cells are more resistant to NK activity than are parental or poorly metastatic cells.[73-75]

B. Influence of NK Modulation on Formation of Metastases

If NK cells play an important role in inhibiting the formation of metastases, then one would expect that a given tumor would metastasize better in an NK-depressed host and less well in a host with augmented NK activity. This hypothesis has been tested by examining the metastatic potential of various experimental tumors in mice with low NK activity due to age-related variations[7,19,20,76-79] or the beige mutation.[80] Mice with low levels of NK activity were found to have a higher incidence of metastases following challenge with metastatic tumors.[27,80-82] NK activity can also be depressed by a variety of agents with differing degrees of selectivity. The chemotherapeutic drug cyclophosphamide (Cy) efficiently decreased NK activity following a single administratin of 100 to 200 mg i.p.[83,84] The same procedure also induced a significant augmentation in the formation of pulmonary metastases and extrapulmonary metastases following i.v. injection of various tumor lines.[27,53] Similarly, depression of NK activity by treatment of mice with β-estradiol,[85,86] anti-asGM-1 serum,[87-93] and anti-NK-1 antisera[94-97] also resulted in increased formation of metastases following subsequent challenge with metastatic tumor cells.

Conversely, numerous BRMs which augment NK activity also increase resistance to formation of metastases.[27,28] These BRMs include *P. acnes,*[77] OK-432,[98] MVE2, poly I:C[99,100] IFN,[101,102] and IL-2[103] among others. However, with all of these BRMs, it has not been possible to unequivocally determine whether the antimetastatic effects of the agents are directly attributable to the augmentation of NK activity or to other, non-NK cell-mediated, effects. It has been particularly difficult to determine which BRM-induced effects are due to NK activity and which are due to activated macrophages. Recently, there have been two approaches to distinguish which effector cell type mediates increased resistance to metastasis following BRM treatment. First, several BRMs have been found to augment NK activity but not macrophage-mediated activity. For example, periodate-oxidized *P. acnes*, which augments NK activity, but fails to augment macrophage-mediated cytotoxicity,[27] has been found to retain the in vivo antimetastatic activity associated with untreated *P. acnes*.[27] Second, both the NK-augmentation and increased resistance to B16 or UV-2237 metastases observed following pretreatment of mice with MVE-2[53] or MTP-PE[54] have been shown to be eliminated by treatment with anti-asGM-1 serum. In contrast, macrophage-mediated activity following these treatments remained largely intact.[53,54,89] Therefore, it appears that a considerable portion of the increased resistance to metastases induced by BRMs is attributable to the augmentation of NK activity.

Additional evidence regarding the relationship between levels of NK activity and resistance to metastasis formation can be found in Chapter 3 and Chapter 8 of these volumes.

Overall, these data strongly support but do not prove the hypothesis that NK cells are active at some stage(s) of the metastatic cascade and thereby inhibit the formation of metastatic foci. The most convincing support for the hypothesis that NK cells are important in host resistance to the formation of metastases would be provided by a demonstration that reconstitution of NK-depressed animals with purified NK cells results in concomitant restoration of this resistance to metastasis formation. Hanna and Burton[96] have demonstrated that the metastasis-enhancing effect of Cy could be reversed by reconstitution of Cy-treated mice with NK-1.2+ spleen cells. Perhaps the best evidence has been provided by Barlozzari et al.,[105] who demonstrated that purified LGL, highly enriched in NK activity and depleted of macrophages and other identifiable cell types, could restore both NK activity in the peripheral blood, as well as antimetastatic resistance,[93] in rats previously treated with anti-asGM-1 serum. These experiments provide convincing evidence that NK cells function as antimetastatic effectors in normal animals.

IV. ROLE OF NK CELLS DURING VARIOUS STAGES OF THE METASTATIC PROCESS

There is no compelling available evidence to implicate NK cells as participating in the control of metastasis at the level of the primary tumor. There are two reasons for this lack of evidence. First, within this compartment there occurs a complex series of events, beginning with the dissociation of individual tumor cells or emboli from the primary tumor, and concluding with successful entry of tumor cells into the vasculature. There is currently no definitive technology available for assessing the role of various effector cells during these events. Second, any antimetastatic effects which would be induced by BRMs in this compartment would be included in the general category of primary tumor therapy. Therefore, we will focus our discussion on NK-mediated events which occur during the intravascular dissemination of tumor cells or their subsequent extravasation into the tissues of target organs.

A. Role of NK Cells During the Intravascular Phase of Metastasis

The preponderance of evidence suggests that the most significant metastasis-inhibiting effects of NK cells occur in the blood stream. The data to support this conclusion have been accumulated in several experimental models in both mice and rats. Peripheral blood of rodents and humans contains a considerable number of NK-active LGL[5,9,104,105] and levels of PBL NK activity has been found to correlate directly with the rate at which i.v.-injected tumor cells are eliminated from the circulation.[27,81,93,105-111] Thus, the rate at which i.v.-injected tumor cells are cleared from the vasculature, conveniently measured in the lung, provides an assay with which to measure NK activity in vivo.[88,112-117] The events measured by this technique are largely intravascular, since the assay measures changes that occur in 1 to 6 hr whereas appreciable extravasation of tumor cells does not occur until at least 4 hr.[1]

Most studies indicating a role for NK cells in the clearance of tumor cells which arrested in the lungs have demonstrated either an association of impaired clearance in animals with innately low or exogenously suppressed NK activity, or an association of accelerated clearance in mice with BRM-augmented NK activity. Riccardi et al.[107] observed that the clearance rate of i.v.-injected RBL-5 tumor cells from lung, liver, and spleen correlated with levels of NK activity in various strains of recipient mice. A strain with low NK activity (SJL) retained ^{125}IdUrd-labeled tumor cells for longer periods of time than did mice with higher levels of NK activity (CBA). These results have been subsequently extended to other strains of mice,[110] including the NK-deficient beige mouse.[81] Conversely, nude mice which generally exhibited higher levels of NK activity than their nu/+ litter-mates, also exhibited accelerated clearance of i.v.-injected tumor cells.[82,111] Cumulatively, these results indicate that NK cells in normal mice contribute to the elimination of tumor cells from the vasculature.

Modulation of NK activity has also been shown to lead to a parallel alteration in the rate at which tumor cells are cleared from the vasculature. For example, the administration of Cy, which impairs NK activity, significantly decreased the rate at which i.v.-injected tumor cells were cleared from the pulmonary vasculature of mice[27,53] and rats.[105] Both NK activity and in vivo tumor cell clearance were restored by reconstitution with spleen cells.[101] Depression of NK activity by administration of the more NK-selective reagents anti-NK 1.1 or anti-asGM-1 to mice,[53,82,95,110] or rats,[105] also decreased the rate of elimination of intravascularly localized tumor cells. Finally Barlozzari et al.[105] have shown that the depression of NK activity and the impairment of tumor clearance induced by anti-asGM-1 serum were concomitantly reconstituted by adoptive transfer with low numbers of highly enriched NK-active LGL. Conversely, Riccardi et al.[107] demonstrated that administration of poly I:C augmented NK activity, and accelerated the rate at which i.v.-injected tumor cells were cleared from the capillary beds of target organs. Others have noted similar effects with other BRMs including *P. acnes,*[27] IFN,[101] or pyran copolymers.[53]

The preceding results suggest that NK cells contribute to prophylaxis of metastasis formation during the blood-borne stage of tumor dissemination in both normal and BRM-treated animals. This hypothesis is supported by several studies which have correlated the NK-dependent intravascular clearance rate of tumor cells with formation of detectable metastatic foci.[27,53,81,82,93,102,105,111] In general, the increased survival of tumor cells in low-NK mice has been paralleled by increased development of metastases following i.v. tumor challenge.[82] Similarly, the impaired tumor cell clearance induced by Cy[27] or anti-asGM-1 serum[53,82,105,111] was accompanied by greatly increased formation of metastases in mice[27,53,82] and rats.[93,105] Furthermore, reconstitution of depressed NK activity and tumor cell clearance by purified LGL coincided with restoration of prophylaxis of metastasis formation.[93,105] Therefore, these results indicate that NK cells exert strong antitumor effects during the intravascular blood-borne phase of tumor metastasis.

B. Role of NK Cells During the Extravasation/Postextravasation Phase of Tumor Metastasis in BRM-Treated Mice

Recent studies have suggested that BRMs can induce NK-mediated antimetastatic resistance not only in the vasculature, but also in various organs during the extravasation/postextravasation stages of metastasis.[53,54] Evidence for this conclusion has come from two types of experiments.

First, as discussed above, the administration of MVE-2 augmented NK activity in the lungs, liver, blood, and spleen, as well as inducing resistance to metastasis formation. A single administration of anti-asGM-1 serum or 100 mg/kg Cy to MVE-2 treated mice depressed the augmented blood and splenic NK levels, but did not appreciably affect the NK activity in the lungs or liver. These same treatments also inhibited the rate at which i.v.-injected tumor cells were cleared from the vasculature in MVE-2 treated mice. However, in spite of this inhibition of blood and splenic NK activity, the antimetastatic effects of MVE-2 were largely retained. Since NK activity in the lungs and liver remained augmented, we postulated that this organ-associated augmentation of NK activity was contributing to the antimetastatic effects of MVE-2. This hypothesis was tested by devising regimen whereby two doses of anti-asGM-1 serum or a higher dose of Cy (200 mg/kg) were used to depress MVE-2 augmented organ-associated NK activity to below the levels in normal, untreated mice. Such abrogation of organ-associated NK activity was found to be associated with loss of MVE-2 induced antimetastatic effects.[54] These results implied that NK cells had an important contribution to the inhibition of tumor cell growth during the extravasation/postextravasation phase of metastasis in local organ compartments.

The second approach was predicated on the postulate that selective augmentation of organ-associated NK activity should be sufficient to induce BRM-mediated antimetastatic effects. Since we made the observation that liposomes incorporating MTP-PE selectively augmented NK activity in the lungs and liver, but not in blood and spleen,[54] we predicted that the antimetastatic activity of liposomes incorporating MTP-PE should be demonstrable in spite of an inability to augment NK activity in the blood. Further, elimination of this augmented organ-association NK activity should coincide with a loss of antimetastatic activity. Our results demonstrated that MTP-PE encapsulated in liposomes preferentially augmented NK activity in the lungs and liver, and concomitantly inhibited the formation of metastases in those organs (Table 1). As predicted, elimination of this augmented NK activity in the lungs and liver by anti-asGM-1 treatment also resulted in increased metastatic formation.[54] It must be emphasized that both MVE-2, or MTP-PE encapsulated in liposomes, prime[89,112] or activate[54] macrophages for tumoricidal activity, respectively. However, under the treatment regimens employed, macrophage-mediated antitumor effects mediated by BRMS are not impaired by the NK depressive anti-asGM-1 serum.[51,53,54,89]

Cumulatively, these results indicate that the role of NK cells in the prophylactic antimetastatic effects of BRMs is not totally limited to the intravascular phase of tumor metastasis. Rather, the results indicate that BRMs also can induce antimetastatic effects later in the metastatic process and that these effects are dependent on augmented NK activity in the various organs.

V. POTENTIAL ROLE OF NK CELLS IN TREATMENT OF PRE-EXISTENT METASTASES

In addition to the prophylactic antimetastatic affects induced by BRMs in local sites of metastasis formation, it may be useful to consider the potential role of NK cells in later events in the treatment of pre-existent metastases. Most BRMs which augment NK activity have been reported to have their most significant effects on tumor growth when administered prior to tumor injection.[27] This has led to the conclusion that NK cells are important in protecting against the establishment of metastases, and that the major antimetastatic role of NK augmentation in tumor-bearing hosts may be the inhibition of formation of secondary or tertiary metastases.[27] This hypothesis is consistent with the observation that distant metastases may reoccur less frequently in patients with high NK activity than those with low NK activity.[113]

However, there have been several considerations which prompt re-evaluation of pre-

Table 1

RELATIONSHIP OF NK ACTIVITY IN VARIOUS ANATOMICAL
COMPARTMENTS AND IN VIVO CLEARANCE OF TUMOR CELLS
TO FORMATION OF METASTASES IN THE LUNGS AND LIVER[a]

In vivo treatment[b]	Formation of metastases	Correlation between formation of metastases and changes in: NK activity Lung/liver	Blood/spleen	In vivo tumor cell clearance
Anti-asGM₁ (low or high dose)	↑	Yes	Yes	Yes
MVE-2	↓	Yes	Yes	Yes
Anti-asGM₁ (low dose) + MVE-2	↓	Yes	No	No
Anti-asGM₁ (high dose) + MVE-2	↑	Yes	Yes	Yes
Cy (low or high dose)	↑	Yes	Yes	Yes
Cy (low dose) + MVE-2	↓	Yes	ND	No
Cy (high dose) + MVE-2	↑	Yes	Yes	Yes
MTP-PE in liposomes	↓	Yes	No	ND
MTP-PE in liposomes + Anti-asGM₁	↑	Yes	Yes	Yes

[a] Abbreviations used include: Anti-asGM₁, anti-asialo GM₁ serum; MVE-2, maleic anhydride divinyl ether; Cy, cyclophosphamide; MTP-PE, muramyl tripeptide-phosphatidylethanolamine; ND, not done.

[b] Details of experimental protocols used to obtain this summary are found in References 58 and 59.

vious attempts at immunotherapy by BRM-induced augmentation of NK activity *in situ*. First, there have been several studies which demonstrated the presence of NK cells in primary tumors.[114-117] These results imply that NK cells may also infiltrate metastases, where their activity may be augmented by BRMs. Secondly, most studies have been performed by administering a single dose of BRM at some time after establishment of metastatic foci.[27] Under these conditions, NK activity only remains augmented for several days.[27,59,61,62] More sustained augmentation of NK activity would be desirable in order to rigorously test the immunotherapeutic potential of NK cells. In fact, sustained activation was also required to achieve regression of pulmonary metastases by alveolar macrophages.[118] Third, in situations where NK-augmenting BRMs have been repeatedly administered, there has often developed a hyporesponsivenss to augmentation of NK activity. Fourth, BRMs generally augment the activity of other effector cells including macrophages. Therefore, it is difficult to definitively separate NK-mediated BRM-induced immunotherapeutic effects from those mediated by macrophages or other effector cells. Fifth, it has become increasingly clear that BRMs do not augment NK activity equally in all anatomical compartments. This implies that NK-mediated BRM-induced antitumor effects might not be equally efficient against tumors in diverse anatomical locations, and that different BRMs which induce augmentation of NK activity in different compartments should be rigorously tested against established metastases in those compartments where their NK-augmenting effects are greatest.

An alternative approach to *in situ* activation for determining the potential role of NK cells against pre-existent metastases involves adoptive immunotherapy by purified populations of NK cells. Reynolds et al.[67] have recently characterized the distribution patterns of radiolabeled rat blood-derived LGL following i.v. or i.p. transfer into normal recipients. These results have demonstrated that the adoptively transferred LGL rapidly localize in several organs following i.v. transfer, whereas most of the cells are retained in the peritoneal cavity following i.p. transfer. These results imply that a model could be constructed to assess the regional therapeutic efficiency of LGL transferred to a localized site of tumor growth, such as occurs frequently in the peritoneal cavity of patients with ovarian cancer.

Further studies will be required to determine whether i.v. transferred LGL can "home" to tumors or metastases in distant sites. Reconstitution of resistance to metastases has been achieved with both purified LGL[93] as well as with IL-2-dependent, in vitro grown NK cell clones.[119] However, rigorous evidence for the effects of these cell types on pre-existent metastatic disease is limited.

Additional observations have also shown that IL-2-grown splenic lymphocytes, which have significant cytotoxic activity against a variety of tumors, also are capable of eradicating pre-existent lung micrometastases[120] following i.v. transfer to tumor-bearing mice. However, it must be noted that while lymphocytes grown in IL-2 for more than several days exhibit enhanced cytotoxic activity, the target cell specificity of these cells is broader than that normally expressed by NK-active LGL.[22] This observation has resulted in some controversy over whether this type of cytolytic activity should actually be designated as NK activity, and whether the IL-2-grown cytolytic cells arise from LGL or non-LGL. Grimm et al.[121] have presented evidence that IL-2 propagated LAK cells can arise from non-NK cells, and that these cells possess T-cell markers not found on NK cells. Conversely, Itoh et al.[24] have recently reported that human lymphocytes with NK activity and expressing the NK-associated Leu-11 phenotype can give rise to broadly cytotoxic cells following growth in IL-2. Therefore, the simplest way to interpret these data is that both LGL and non-LGL can respond to IL-2 by proliferation and expression of broad tumoricidal activity, and that NK cells may contribute to the therapeutic effects of rIL-2 stimulated cytotoxic cells. Ettinghausen, et al.,[122] have reported that in vivo administration of human recombinant IL-2 stimulated proliferation of Thy 1.2 positive lymphocytes in many organs, including lung and liver. We have previously demonstrated that LGL isolated from BRM-treated mice were strongly Thy 1.2 positive.[10] Therefore NK cells may contribute to the therapeutic effects associated with administration of rIL-2.

Overall, it is clear that NK cells play an important role in inhibiting the formation of metastases. However, their potential role in the therapy of established metastases remains unclear. Recent advances in isolating, characterizing, and growing NK cells in vitro, combined with a better understanding of how long and where NK activity is augmented by BRMs, will provide a more definitive understanding of the potential for NK cells in BRM-induced immunotherapy.

VI. SUMMARY AND PERSPECTIVES

The major role of NK cells in inhibiting metastases in normal animals probably occurs in the vascular compartment of the metastatic cascade. However, the administration of BRMs increases NK-mediated resistance to metastases by not only increasing NK-mediated intravascular activity but also by inducing organ-associated NK cells in the target organs where metastases are ultimately seeded. It has become apparent that sustained augmentation of organ-associated NK activity requires a better understanding of the dynamic effects of BRMs on systemic and compartmentalized levels of NK activity. This is necessary to circumvent the development of hyporesponsiveness to augmentation of NK activity at sites of tumor growth, which can occur following multiple treatments with some BRMs. Further, an understanding of these events is critical to "targeting" NK-mediated BRM therapy to tumors in selected organs. This approach involves testing the ability of NK cells to inhibit the growth of pre-existing metastases in the organ sites preferentially infiltrated by LGL following BRM administration. Conceivably, these preferential sites of LGL localization may differ depending on the BRM administered, and therefore this aspect of BRM treatment should be considered when investigating NK-mediated antitumor effects. Furthermore, since most BRMs affect non-NK cells as well as NK cells, the possible effects of such cells on down-regulation of NK activity in local compartments of tumor growth should not be over-looked. Thus, successful BRM therapy may depend not only on the ability to augment the antitumor effects of the relevant effector cells, but also on the ability to limit down-regulation by other cell types.

Another approach to NK-mediated treatment of metastatic disease, which contrasts to *in situ* augmentation of NK activity, would be adoptive therapy with NK cells. Currently, the only way to obtain sufficient NK cells for these studies is to propagate cells in IL-2. This approach may be most effective for therapy of peritoneal disease[123] or disease in specific organs[124] because the IL-2-cultured cells do not appear to distribute with the same pattern as normal lymphocytes.[125] Therefore, adoptive therapy of metastases may be subject to some of the same practical restrictions as *in situ* modulation NK activity in that certain types of tumors in several defined anatomical locations may be the most likely candidates for successful BRM treatment.

Overall, it is clear that NK cells, especially after augmentation with BRMs, can lyse a broad spectrum of tumor cells in vitro and in vivo. The potential of these cells to control pre-existing metastases should become more clearly understood in the next several years as approaches which maximize the interaction between NK cells and tumor foci are elucidated.

REFERENCES

1. Fidler, I. J., Gersten, D. M., and Hart, I. R., The biology of cancer invasion and metastasis, *Adv. Cancer Res.*, 28, 149, 1978.
2. Poste, G. and Fidler, I. J., The pathogenesis of cancer metastasis, *Nature (London)*, 283, 139, 1980.
3. Talmadge, J. E., The selective nature of metastasis, *Cancer Met. Rev.*, 2, 25, 1983.
4. Koren, H. S. and Herberman, R. B., Natural killing — present and future (summary of workshop on natural killer cells), *J. Natl. Cancer Inst.*, 70, 785, 1983.
5. Timonen, T. and Saksela, E., Isolation of human natural killer cells by discontinuous gradient centrifugation, *J. Immunol. Methods*, 36, 285, 1980.
6. Timonen, T., Reynolds, C. W., Ortaldo, J. R., and Herberman, R. B., Isolation of human and rat natural killer cells, *J. Immunol. Methods*, 51, 269, 1982.
7. Reynolds, C. W., Timonen, T. T., and Herberman, R. B., Natural killer (NK) cell activity in the rat. I. Isolation and characterization of the effector cells, *J. Immunol.*, 127, 282, 1981.
8. Kumagai, K., Itoh, K., Suzkui, R., Hinuma, S., and Saitoh, F., Studies of murine large granular lymphocytes. I. Identification as effector cells in NK and K cytotoxicities, *J. Immunol.*, 129, 388, 1982.
9. Itoh, K., Suzuki, R., Umezu, Y., Hanaumi, K., and Kumagai, K., Studies of murine large granular lymphocytes. II. Tissue, strain, and age distribution of LGL and LAL, *J. Immunol.*, 129, 395, 1982.
10. Wiltrout, R. H., Mathieson, B. J., Talmadge, J. E., Reynolds, C. W., Zhang, S.-R., Herberman, R. B., and Ortaldo, J. R., Augmentation of organ-associated NK activity by biological response modifiers: isolation and characterization of large granular lymphocytes from the liver, *J. Exp. Med.*, 160, 1431, 1984.
11. Tagliabue, A., Befus, A. D., Clark, D. A., and Bienenstock, J., Characteristics of natural killer cells in the murine intestinal epithelium and lamina propria, *J. Exp. Med.*, 155, 1785, 1982.
12. Leventon, G. S., Kulkarni, S. S., Meistrich, M. L., Newland, J. R., and Zanden, A. R., Isolation of murine small bowell intraepithelial lymphocytes, *J. Immunol. Methods*, 63, 35, 1983.

13. Stein-Streilein, J., Bennett, M., Mann, D., and Kumar, V., Natural killer cells in mouse lung: surface phenotype, target preference, and response to local influenza virus infection, *J. Immunol.*, 131, 2699, 1983.
14. Kaneda, K., Dan, C., and Wake, K., Pit cells as natural killer cells, *Biomed. Res.*, 4, 567, 1983.
15. Lukomska, B., Olzewski, W. L., and Engeset, A., Rat liver contains a distinct blood-borne population of NK cells resistant to anti-asialo GM₁ antiserum, *Immunol. Lett.*, 6, 277, 1983.
16. Ward, J. M., Argilan, F., and Reynolds, C. W., Immunoperoxidase localization of large granular lymphocytes in normal tissues and lesions of athymic nude rats, *J. Immunol.*, 131, 132, 1983.
17. Kasai, M., Iwamori, M., Nagai, Y., Okumura, K., and Tada, T., A glycolipid on the surface of mouse natural killer cells, *Eur. J. Immunol.*, 10, 175, 1980.
18. Reynolds, C. W., Sharrow, S. O., Ortaldo, J. R., and Herberman, R. B., Natural killer activity in the rat. II. Analysis of surface antigens on LGL by flow cytometry, *J. Immunol.*, 127, 2204, 1981.
19. Herberman, R. B., Nunn, M. E., and Lavrin, D. H., Natural cytotoxic reactivity of mouse lymphoid cells against syngeneic and allogeneic tumors. I. Distribution of reactivity and specificity, *Int. J. Cancer*, 16, 216, 1975.
20. Herberman, R. B. and Holden, H. T., Natural cell-mediated immunity, *Adv. Cancer Res.*, 27, 305, 1978.
21. Reynolds, C. W., Timonen, T. T., Holden, H. T., Hansen, C. T., and Herberman, R. B., Natural killer (NK) cell activity in the rat. Analysis of effector cell morphology and effects of interferon on NK cell function in the athymic (nude) rat, *Eur. J. Immunol.*, 12, 577, 1982.
22. Allavena, P. and Ortaldo, J. R., Characteristics of human NK clones: target specificity and phenotype, *J. Immunol.*, 132, 2363, 1984.
23. Ortaldo, J. R., Mason, A. T., Gerard, J. P., Henderson, L. E., Farrar, W., Hopkins, R. F., III, Herberman, R. B., and Rabin, H., Effects of natural and recombinant IL-2 on regulation of IFN gamma production and natural killer activity: lack of involvement of the Tac antigen for these immunoregulatory effects, *J. Immunol.*, 133, 779, 1984.
24. Itoh, K., Tilden, A. B., Kumagai, K., and Balch, C. M., Leu-11⁺ lymphocytes with natural killer (NK) activity are precursors of recombinant interleukin 2 (rIL2)-induced activated killer (AK) cells, *J. Immunol.*, 134, 802, 1985.
25. Djeu, J. Y., Heinbaugh, J. A., Holden, H. T., and Herberman, R. B., Augmentation of mouse natural killer cell activity by interferon and interferon inducers, *J. Immunol.*, 122, 175, 1979.
26. Ortaldo, J. R., Mason, A., Rehnbey, E., Moscheru, J., Kelder, B., Pestka, S., and Herberman, R. B., Effects of recombinant and hybrid recombinant human leukocyte interferon on cytotoxic activity of natural killer cells, *J. Biol. Chem.*, in press, 1985.
27. Hanna, N., Role of natural killer cells in control of cancer metastasis, *Cancer Met. Rev.*, 1, 45, 1982.
28. Wiltrout, R. H., Talmadge, J. E., and Herberman, R. B., Augmentation of natural killer activity by biological response modifiers: potential role in prevention and treatment of metastatic disease, *Adv. Immun. Cancer Ther.*, in press.
29. Herberman, R. B., *Natural Cell Mediated Immunity Against Tumors*, Academic Press, New York, 1980, pp. 1321.
30. Herberman, R. B., NK *Cells and Other Natural Effector Cells*, Academic Press, New York, 1982, pp. 1566.
31. Trinchieri, G. and Santoli, D., Anti-viral activity induced by culturing lymphocytes with tumor-derived or virus-transformed cells. Enhancement of natural killer activity by interferon and antagonistic inhibition of susceptibility of target cells to lysis, *J. Exp. Med.*, 147, 1314, 1978.
32. Trinchieri, G., Santoli, D., Dee, R. R., and Knowles, B. B., Antiviral activity by culturing lymphocytes with tumor-derived or virus-transformed cells: identification of the human effector lymphocyte subpopulation, *J. Exp. Med.*, 147, 1299, 1978.
33. Welsh, R. M., NK cells and interferon, *CRC Rev.*, in press.
34. Ortaldo, J. R., and Herberman, R. B., Augmentation of natural killer activity, in *Immunobiology of Natural Killer Cells*, Lotzova, E. and Herberman, R. B., Eds., CRC Press, Boca Raton, Fla., in press, 1985.
35. Henney, C. S., Kurabayashi, K., Kern, D. E., and Gillis, S., Interleukin-2 augments natural killer cell activity, *Nature (London)*, 291, 335, 1981.
36. Ortaldo, J. R., Gerard, J. P., Henderson, L. E., Neubauer, R. H., and Rabin, H., Responsiveness of purified natural killer cells to pure interleukin-2 (IL-2), in *Interleukins, Lymphokines and Cytokines*, Oppenheim, J. J. and Rabin, H., eds., Academic Press, New York, 1983, pp. 63.
37. Mathews, P. M., Froelich, C. J., Sibbit, W. L., and Bankhurst, A. D., Enhancement of natural cytotoxicity by β-endorphin, *J. Immunol.*, 130, 1658, 1983.
38. Faith, R. E., Liang, H. J., Murgo, A. J., and Plotnikoff, N. P., Neuro-immunomodulation with enkaphalins: enhancement of human natural killer (NK) cell activity *in vitro*, *Clin. Immunol. Immunopathol.*, 31, 412, 1984.

39. Tolcott, P. A., Exon, J. H., and Koller, L. D., Alteration of natural killer cell-mediated cytotoxicity in rats treated with selenium, diethylnitrosamine, and ethylnitrosourea, *Cancer Lett.*, 23, 313, 1984.
40. Shitara, K., Ichimura, O., Mitsuno, T., and Osawa, T., Natural killer (NK) cell activating factor released from murine thymocytes stimulated with an antitumor streptococcal preparation, OK-432, *J. Immunol.*, 134, 1039, 1985.
41. Brunda, M. J., Herberman, R. B., and Holden, H. T., Antibody-induced augmentation of murine natural killer cell activity, *Int. J. Cancer*, 27, 205, 1981.
42. Welsh, R. M., Cytotoxic cells induced during lymphocyte choriomeningitis virus infection in mice. I. Characterization of natural killer cell induction, *J. Exp. Med.*, 148, 163, 1978.
43. Welsh, R. M., Zinkernagel, R. M., and Hallenbeck, L. A., Cytotoxic cells induced during lymphocytic choriomeningitis virus infection of mice. II. Specificities of the natural killer cells, *J. Immunol.*, 122, 475, 1979.
44. Biron, C. A. and Welsh, R. M., Proliferation and role of natural killer cells during viral infection, in *NK Cells and Other Natural Effector Cells*, Herberman, R. B., ed., Academic Press, New York, 1982, pp. 493.
45. Bukowski, J. F., Biron, C. A., and Welsh, R. M., Elevated natural killer cell-mediated cytotoxicity, plasma interferon and tumor cells rejection in mice persistently infected with lymphocytic choriomeningitis, *J. Immunol.*, 131, 991, 1983.
46. Bukowski, J. F., Woda, B. A., Habu, S., Okumura, K., and Welsh, R. M., Natural killer cell depletion enhances virus synthesis and virus-induced hepatitis *in vivo*, *J. Immunol.*, 131, 1531, 1983.
47. Niederkorn, J. Y., Brieland, J. K., and Mayhew, E., Enhanced natural killer cell activity in experimental murine enceophalitozoonosis, *Infect. Immun.*, 41, 302, 1983.
48. Wiltrout, R. H., Salup, R. R., Twilley, T. A., and Talmadge, J. E., Immunomodulation of NK activity by polyribonucleotides, *J. Biological Resp. Mod.*, 4, 512, 1985.
49. Wiltrout, R. H., Reynolds, C. W., Ortaldo, J. R., Salup, R., and Talmadge, J. E., Augmentation of NK activity in lungs and livers of mice by biological response modifiers (BRMs); application to immunotherapy by BRMs, in *Proc. 14th Int. Congress Chemother.*, University of Tokyo Press, 955, 1985.
50. Wiltrout, R. H., Salup, R. R., and Talmadge, J. E., Augmentation of liver-associated NK activity by OK-432, Tokyo, *Excerpta Med.*, in press,
51. Zhang, S. R., Urias, P. L., Twilley, T. A., Talmadge, J. E., Herberman, R. B., and Wiltrout, R. H., Augmentation of tumoricidal activity mediated by NK cells and macrophages in the livers of mice following treatment with biological response modifiers, *Cancer Immunol. Immunother.*, 21, 19, 1986.
52. Talmadge, J. E., Herberman, R. B., Chirigos, M. A., Schneider, M. A., Adams, J. S., Phillips, H., Thurman, G. B., Varesio, L., Long, C. A., Oldham, R. K., and Wiltrout, R. H., Augmentation or induction of a hyporesponsivenss of murine NK activity by various classes of immunomodulators including recombinant interferons and interleukin 2, *J. Immunol.*, 135, 2483, 1985.
53. Wiltrout, R. H., Herberman, R. B., Chirigos, M. A., Ortaldo, J. R., Green, K. M., Jr., and Talmadge, J. E., Role of NK cells in lung and liver in decreased formation of experimental metastases, *J. Immunol.*, 134, 4267, 1985.
54. Talmadge, J. E., Schneider, M., Collins, M., Phillips, H., Herberman, R. B., and Wiltrout, R. H., Augmentation of NK cell activity in tissue specific sites by liposomes incorporating MTP-PE, *J. Immunol.*, 135, 1477, 1985.
55. Hurme, M., Silvennoinen, O., and Renkonen, R., Highly increased natural killer cell number and lytic activity in the murine peripheral blood and lungs after interferon induction in vivo, *Scand. J. Immunol.*, 20, 371, 1984.
56. Bruley-Rosset, M. and Rappaport, H., Natural killer cell activity and spontaneous development of lymphoma: effects of single and multiple injections into young and aged C57B1/6 mice, *Int. J. Cancer*, 31, 381, 1983.
57. Maluish, A. E., Ortaldo, J. R., Conlon, J. C., Sherwin, S. A., Leavitt, R., Strong, D. M., Weirnik, P., Oldham, R. K., and Herberman, R. B., Depression of natural killer cytotoxicity following in vivo administration of recombinant leukocyte interferon, *J. Immunol.*, 131, 503, 1983.
58. Huddlestone, J. R., Merigan, T. C., and Oldstone, M. B. A., Induction and kinetics of natural killer cells in humans following interferon therapy, *Nature (London)*, 282, 417, 1979.
59. Talmadge, J. E., Maluish, A. E., Collins, M., Schneider, M., Herberman, R. B., Oldham, R. K., and Wiltrout, R. H., Immunomodulation and antitumor effects of MVE-2 in mice, *J. Biol. Resp. Modif.*, 3, 634, 1984.
60. Piccoli, M., Saito, T., and Chirigos, M. A., Bimodal effects of MVE-2 on cytotoxic activity of natural killer cell and macrophage-mediated tumoricidal activities, *Int. J. Immunopharmacol.*, 6, 569, 1984.
61. Hanna, N., Regulation of natural killer cell activation: implementation for the control of tumor metastasis, *Nat. Immun. Cell Growth Reg.*, 3, 22, 1984.

62. Savary, C. A. and Lotzova, E., Suppression of natural killer cell cytotoxicity be splenocytes from *Corynebacterium parvum*-injected, bone marrow tolerant and infant mice, *J. Immunol.*, 120, 239, 1978.
63. Santoni, A., Riccardi, C., Barlozzari, T., and Herberman, R. B., *C. parvum*-induced suppressor cells for mouse NK activity, in *NK Cells and Other Natural Effector Cells*, Herberman, R. B., Ed., Academic Press, New York, 1982, pp. 519.
64. Biron, C. A., Turgiss, L. R., and Welsh, R. M., Increase in NK cell number and turnover rate during acute virus infection, *J. Immunol.*, 131, 1539, 1983.
65. Biron, C. A. and Welsh, R. M., Blastogenesis of natural killer cells during viral infection *in vivo*, *J. Immunol.*, 129, 2788, 1982.
66. Santoni, A., Piccoli, M., Ortaldo, J. R., Mason, L., Wiltrout, R. H., and Herberman, R. B., Changes in number and density of large granular lymphocytes upon *in vivo* augmentation of mouse natural killer activity, *J. Immunol.*, 134, 2799, 1985.
67. Reynolds, C. W., Denn, III, A. C., Barlozzari, T., Wiltrout, R. H., and Herberman, R. B., Natural killer activity in the rat. IV. Distribution of large granular lymphocytes (LGL) following intravenous and intraperitoneal transfer, *Cell. Immunol.*, 86, 371, 1984.
68. Gorelik, E., Feldman, M., and Segal, S., Selection of 3LL tumor subline resistant to natural effector cells concomitantly selected for increased metastatic potency, *Cancer Immunol. Immunother.*, 12, 105, 1982.
69. Brodt, P., Feldman, M., and Segal, S., Differences in the metastatic potential of two sublines of tumor 3LL selected for resistance to natural NK-like effector cells, *Cancer Immunol. Immunother.*, 16, 109, 1983.
70. Poupon, M.-F., Judde, J. G., Pot-Deprun, J., Sweeney, F., and Lespinats, G., Variable susceptibility to NK activity of cloned cell lines derived from a primary rat rhabdomyosarcoma: relationship to metastatic potential, *Br. J. Cancer*, 48, 75, 1983.
71. Hanna, N. and Fidler, I., Relationship between metastatic potential and resistance to natural killer cell-mediated cytotoxicity in three murine tumor systems, *J. Natl. Cancer Inst.*, 66, 1183, 1981.
72. Thorgeirsson, U. P., Turpeenniemi-Hujanen, T., Williams, J. E., Westin, E. H., Heilman, C. A., Talmadge, J. E., and Liotta, L. A., Metastatic phenotype is expressed by NIH 3T3 cells transfected with human tumor DNA containing the N-ras oncogene, *Mol. Cell. Biol.*, in press, 5:1985.
73. Gorelik, E., Fogel, M., Feldman, M., and Segal, S., Differences in resistance of metastatic tumor cells and cells from local tumor growth to cytotoxicity of natural killer cells, *J. Natl. Cancer Inst.*, 63, 1397, 1979.
74. Brooks, C. G., Flannery, G. A., Willmott, N., Austin, E. B., Kenwrick, S., and Baldwin, R. W., Tumor cells in metastatic deposits with; altered sensitivity to natural killer cells, *Int. J. Cancer*, 28, 191, 1981.
75. Nestel, F. P., Casson, P. R., Wiltrout, R. H., and Kerbel, R. S., Alterations in sensitivity to non-specific cell-mediated lysis associated with tumor progression, *J. Natl. Cancer Inst.*, 73, 483, 1984.
76. Kiessling, R., Klein, E., and Wigzell, H., Natural killer cells in the mouse. A. Cytotoxic cells with specificity for mouse Moloney leukemia cells. Specificity and distribution according to genotype, *Eur. J. Immunol.*, 5, 112, 1975.
77. Hanna, N., Expression of metastatic potential of tumor cells in young nude mice is correlated with low levels of natural killer cell-mediated cytotoxicity, *Int. J. Cancer*, 26, 675, 1980.
78. Kiessling, R. and Wigzell, H., An analysis of the murine NK cells as to the structure, function, and biological relevance, *Immunol. Rev.*, 44, 165, 1979.
79. Herberman, R. B., Djeu, J. R., Kay, H. D., Ortaldo, J. R., Riccardi, C., Bonnard, G. D., Holden, H. T., Fagnani, R., Santoni, A., and Pucetti, P., Natural killer cells: characteristics and regulation of activity, *Immunol. Rev.*, 44, 43, 1979.
80. Roder, J. and Duwe, A., The beige mutation in the mouse selectivity impairs natural killer cell function, *Nature (London)*, 278, 451, 1979.
81. Talmadge, J., Meyers, K., Prieur, D., and Starkey, J., Role of NK cells in tumor growth and metastasis in beige mice, *Nature (London)*, 284, 622, 1980.
82. Gorelik, E., Wiltrout, R. H., Okumura, K., Habu, S., and Herberman, R. B., Role of NK cells in the control of metastatic spread and growth of tumor cells in mice, *Int. J. Cancer*, 30, 107, 1982.
83. Mantovani, A., Luini, W., Peri, G., Vecchi, A., and Spreafico, F., Effect of chemotherapeutic agents on natural cell-mediated cytotoxicity in mice, *J. Natl. Cancer Inst.*, 61, 1255, 1978.
84. Djeu, J. Y., Heinbaugh, J. A., Vieira, W. D., Holden, H. T., and Herberman, R. B., The effect of immunopharmacological agents on mouse natural cell-mediated cytotoxicity and on its augmentation by poly I:C, *Immunopharmacology*, 1, 231, 1979.
85. Seaman, W. E., Blackman, M. A., Gindhart, T. D., Roubina, J. R., Loeb, J. M., and Talal, N., β-estradiol reduces natural killer cells in mice, *J. Immunol.*, 121, 2193, 1978.
86. Hanna, N. and Schneider, M., Enhancement of tumor metastasis and suppression of natural killer cell activity by β-estradiol treatment, *J. Immunol.*, 130, 974, 1983.

87. Kasai, M., Iwamori, M., Nagai, Y., Okumura, K., and Tada, T., A glycolipid on the surface of mouse natural killer cells, *Eur. J. Immunol.,* 10, 175, 1980.
88. Beck, B. N., Gillis, S., and Henney, C. S., Display of the neutral glycolipid ganglio-N-tetraosylceramide (asialo-GM₁) and cells of the natural killer and T cell lineages, *Transplantation,* 33, 118, 1982.
89. Wiltrout, R. H., Santoni, A., Peterson, E. S., Knott, D. C., Overton, W. R., Herberman, R. B., and Holden, H. T., Reactivity of anti-asialo GM₁ serum with tumoricidal and non-tumoricidal mouse macrophages, *J. Leuk. Biol.,* 37, 597, 1985.
90. Habu, S., Fukui, H., Shimamura, K., Kasai, M., Nagai, Y., Okumura, K., and Tamaoki, N., In vivo effects of anti-asialo GM₁. I. Reduction of NK activity and enhancement of transplanted tumor growth in nude mice, *J. Immunol.,* 127, 34, 1981.
91. Saijo, N., Ozaki, A., Beppu, Y., Takahashi, K., Fujita, J., Sasaki, Y., Nomori, H., Kimata, M., Shimizu, E., and Hoshi, A., Analysis of metastatic spread and growth of tumor cells in mice with depressed natural killer activity by anti-asialo GM₁ antibody or anticancer agents, *J. Cancer Res. Clin. Oncol.,* 107, 157, 1984.
92. Salup, R., Herberman, R. B., and Wiltrout, R. H., Role of natural killer activity in development of spontaneous metastases in murine renal cancer, *J. Urol.,* 134, 1236, 1985.
93. Barlozzari, T., Leonhardt, J., Wiltrout, R. H., Herberman, R. B., and Reynolds, C. W., Direct evidence for the role of NK cells in the inhibition of tumor metastasis, *J. Immunol.,* 134, 2793, 1985.
94. Glimcher, L., Shen, F. W., and Cantor, H., Identification of a cell-surface antigen selectively expressed on the natural killer cell, *J. Exp. Med.,* 145, 1, 1977.
95. Pollock, S. and Hallenbeck, L. A., In vivo reduction of NK activity with anti-NK1 serum: direct evaluation of NK cells in tumor clearance, *Int. J. Cancer,* 29, 203, 1982.
96. Hanna, N. and Burton, R., Definitive evidence that (NK) cells inhibit experimental tumor metastasis in vivo, *J. Immunol.,* 127, 1754, 1981.
97. Burton, R. C., Bartlett, S. O., Kumar, V., and Luinn, H. J., Studies on natural killer (NK) cells. II. Serologic evidence for heterogeneity of murine NK cells, *J. Immunol.,* 127, 1864, 1981.
98. Ishida, N., Hoshino, T., and Uchida, A., A streptococcal preparation as a potent biological response modifier OK-432, Tokyo, *Excerpta Med.,* 1983.
99. Talmadge, J. E., Adams, J., Phillips, H., Collins, M., Lenz, B., Schneider, M., and Chirigos, M. A., Immunotherapeutic potential in murine tumor models of polyinosinic:polycytidylic acid and poly L-lysine solubilized by carboxymethylcellulose, *Cancer Res.,* 45, 1066, 1985.
100. Talmadge, J. E., Adams, J., Phillips, H., Collins, M., Lenz, B., Schneider, M., Wiltrout, R. H., and Chirigos, M. A., Immunodulatory effects of poly ICLC in mice, *Cancer Res.,* 45, 1058, 1985.
101. Brunda, M. J., Rosenbaum, D., and Stern, L., Inhibition of experimentally-induced murine metastases by recombinant alpha interferon: correlation between the modulatory effect of interferon treatment on natural killer cell activity and inhibition of metastases, *Int. J. Cancer,* 34, 421, 1984.
102. Gresser, I. and Brouty-Boye, D., Inhibition by interferon of preparations of solid malignant tumor and pulmonary metastases in mice, *Nature New Biol.,* 236, 78, 1972.
103. Mule, J. J., Shu, S., Schwarz, S. L., and Rosenberg, S. A., Adoptive immunotherapy of established pulmonary metastases with LAK cells and recombinant Interleukin-2, *Science,* 225, 1487, 1984.
104. Santoni, A., Piccoli, M., Ortaldo, J. R., Mason, L., Wiltrout, R. H., and Herberman, R. B., Changes in number and density of large granular lymphocytes upon in vivo augmentation of mouse natural killer activity, *J. Immunol.,* 134, 2799, 1985.
105. Barlozzari, T., Reynolds, C. W., and Herberman, R. B., In vivo role of natural killer cells: involvement of large granular lymphocytes in the clearance of tumor cells in anti-asialo GM₁-treated rats, *J. Immunol.,* 131, 1024, 1983.
106. Riccardi, C., Barlozzari, T., Santoni, A., Herberman, R. B., and Cesarini, C., Transfer to cyclophosphamide-treated mice of natural killer (NK) cells and *in vivo* natural reactivity against tumors, *J. Immunol.,* 126, 1284, 1981.
107. Riccardi, C., Puccetti, P., Santoni, A., and Herberman, R. B., Rapid *in vivo* assay of mouse NK cell activity, *J. Natl. Cancer Inst.,* 63, 1041, 1979.
108. Riccardi, C., Santoni, A., Barlozzari, T., and Herberman, R. B., Role of NK cells in rapid in vivo clearance of radiolabeled tumor cells, in *Natural Cell-Mediated Immunity Against Tumors,* Herberman, R. B., Ed., Academic Press, New York, 1980, 1121.
109. Riccardi, C., Santoni, A., Barlozzari, T., Puccetti, P., and Herberman, R. B., *In vivo* natural reactivity of mice against tumor cells, *Int. J. Cancer,* 25, 475, 1980.
110. Wiltrout, R. H., Gorelik, E., Brunda, M. J., Holden, H. T., and Herberman, R. B., Assessment of *in vivo* natural antitumor resistance and lymphocyte migration in mice: comparison of ¹²⁵I-iododeoxyuridine with ¹¹¹Indium-oxine and ⁵¹Chromium as cell labels, *Cancer Immunol. Immunother.,* 14, 172, 1983.
111. Hanna, N. and Fidler, I. J., The role of natural killer cells in the destruction of circulating tumor emboli, *J. Natl. Cancer Inst.,* 65, 801, 1980.

112. Adams, D. O., Johnson, W. J., Marino, P. A., and Dean, J. H., Effect of pyran co-polymer on activation of murine macrophages: evidence for incomplete activation of functional markers, *Cancer Res.,* 43, 3633, 1983.
113. Hersey, P., Edwards, A., McCorthy, W., and Milton, G., Tumor-related changes and prognostic significance of natural killer cell activity in melanoma patients, in *NK Cells and Other Natural Effector Cells,* Herberman, R. B., Ed., Academic Press, New York, 1982, pp. 1167.
114. Eremin, O., Coombs, R. R. A., and Ashby, J., Lymphocytes infiltrating human breast cancer lack K-cell activity and show low levels of NK-cell activity, *Br. J. Cancer,* 44, 166, 1981.
115. Mantovani, A., Allavena, P., Sessa, C., Bolis, G., and Mangioni, C., Natural killer activity of lymphoid cells isolated from human ascitic ovarian tumors, *Int. J. Cancer,* 25, 573, 1980.
116. Introna, M. and Mantovani, A., Natural killer cells in human solid tumors, *Cancer Met. Rev.,* 2, 337, 1983.
117. Gerson, J. M., Systemic and in situ natural killer activity in tumor-bearing mice and patients with cancer, in *Natural Cell-Mediated Immunity Against Tumors,* Herberman, R. B., Ed., Academic Press, New York, 1980, pp. 1047.
118. Fidler, I. J., Therapy of spontaneous metastases by intravenous injection of liposomes containing lymphokines, *Science,* 208, 1469, 1980.
119. Warner, S. F. and Dennert, G., Effects of a cloned line with NK activity on bone marrow transplants, tumor development, and metastases, *in vivo, Nature (London),* 300, 31, 1982.
120. Mule, J. J., Shu, S., Schwarz, S. L., and Rosenberg, S. A., Adoptive immunotherapy of established pulmonary metastases with LAK cells and recombinant Interleukin-2, *Science,* 225, 1487, 1984.
121. Grimm, E. A., Mazumder, A., Zhang, H. Z., and Rosenberg, S. A., Lymphokine-activated killer cell phenomenon. Lysis of natural killer-resistant fresh solid tumor cells by interleukin 2-activated autologous human peripheral blood lymphocytes, *J. Exp. Med.,* 155, 1823, 1982.
122. Ettinghausen, S. E., Lipford III, E. H., Mule, J. J., and Rosenberg, S. A., Systemic administration of recombinant interleukin 2 stimulates in vivo lymphoid cell proliferation in tissues, *J. Immunol.,* 135, 1488, 1985.
123. Salup, R. R. and Wiltrout, R. H., Treatment of adenocarcinoma in the peritoneum of mice: chemoimmunotherapy with IL-2 stimulated cytotoxic lymphocytes as a model for treatment of minimal residual disease, *Cancer Immun. Immunother.,* 22, 31, 1986.
124. Salup, R. R. and Wiltrout, R. H., Adjuvant immunotherapy of established murine recal cancer by interleukin 2-stimulated cytotoxic lymphocytes, *Cancer Res.,* in press, 1986.
125. Lotze, M. T., Line, B. R., Mathison, D. J., and Rosenberg, S. A., The in vivo distribution of autologous human and murine lymphoid cells in T cell growth factor (TCGF): implications for the adoptive immunotherapy of tumors, *J. Immunol.,* 125, 1487, 1980.
126. Wiltrout, R. H. and Reynolds, C. W., Unpublished observation.
127. Wiltrout, R. H. et al., Manuscript in preparation.

Chapter 10

TREATMENT OF CANCER METASTASIS BY MONONUCLEAR PHAGOCYTES ACTIVATED IN SITU WITH LIPOSOME-ENCAPSU-LATED IMMUNOMODULATORS

W. E. Fogler and I. J. Fidler

TABLE OF CONTENTS

I. INTRODUCTION

Despite advances in surgical excision of primary neoplasms, adjuvant therapy, and improvements in general patient care, most deaths of patients with solid cancers are due to metastases. There are several reasons for the failure to cure metastasis. First, at the time of diagnosis of primary tumors, metastasis may have already occurred, but the lesions are often too small to be detected. Second, the anatomic location of many metastases may limit delivery of therapeutic agents to the lesions without being toxic to normal tissues. The third, and most formidable problem is the heterogeneous nature of malignant neoplasms that leads to the rapid emergence of metastases resistant to conventional therapy.

Recent data from our laboratory and many others indicate that metastases can arise from the nonrandom spread of specialized subpopulations of cells that pre-exist within the primary tumor, that metastases can be clonal in their origin, and that different metastases can originate from different progenitor cells. These data provide an explanation for the clinical observations that even within the same patient, different metastases exhibit different suceptibilities to therapeutic modalities such as chemotherapy. The implication of the varied responses of tumor cells to conventional treatment modalities is that successful therapy of disseminated metastases will have to circumvent the problems of biologic heterogeneity and the development of resistance by tumor cells.

There is now an increasing body of data showing that macrophages activated to the tumoricidal state can fulfill these demanding tasks. In this chapter, we review some of the evidence to support this hypothesis as well as summarize work from our laboratory and many others that deals with the methods to achieve the *in situ* activation of macrophages and the destruction of established metastases.

II. THE INFLUENCE OF HOST IMMUNE STATUS ON THE PATHOGENESIS OF CANCER METASTASIS

The pathogenesis of cancer metastasis depends on the interaction of tumor cells with the host and can be divided into several sequential steps:

1.   Invasion of cells from the primary tumor into the surrounding tissue, with penetration of blood and/or lymph vessels.
2.   Release of single or multiple tumor cell emboli into the circulation.
3.   Arrest of the circulating emboli in the small vascular beds of organs.
4.   Tumor cell extravasation through the vessel wall at the site of arrest and infiltration into adjacent tissue.
5.   Multiplication of tumor cells and the development of vascularized stroma into the new tumor focus.[1-3]

During metastasis, tumor cells come in direct contact with various elements of the immune system, which include macrophages,[4,5] T-lymphocytes,[6,7] NK cells,[8,9] natural cytotoxic cells,[10,11] and neutrophils.[12] The formation of tumor metastases can also be inhibited by soluble effector molecules such as induced or naturally occurring antibodies and complement, tumor necrosis factor,[17,18] lymphotoxin,[19,20] and tumor-derived growth inhibition factor.[21]

Experimental studies on the role of host immunity in cancer metastasis have yielded contradictory results. Highly immunogenic MCA-induced mammary carcinomas did not metastasize in the rat, whereas weakly immunogenic tumors produced extensive metastases. In an experimental metastasis model, tumor cells injected intravenously were arrested primarily in the lungs, and mice bearing small local (subcutaneous) tumors were more resistant to the development of pulmonary metastases than normal mice[23,24] or mice bearing large primary tumors.[24,25] The development of metastatic foci was enhanced by treatment of tumor-bearing mice with antithymocyte serum[26-28] or X-irradiation,[29] and the resistance of normal mice to i.v. challenge with tumor cells was augmented by the transfer of spleen cells[30] or peritoneal cells[28] from immune donors. Serum alone had no effect on the resistance of X-irradiated recipients to i.v. tumor challenge unless normal or immune spleen cells were adoptively transferred into these mice before challenge. Thus, suppression of host immunity was shown to increase the metastatic incidence of malignant mouse neoplasms. Collectively, these results suggest that cellular and humoral immune responses can destroy hematogenously disseminated tumor cells.

That immune suppression can lead to enhanced metastasis is not a generalized phenomenon. In many other tumor systems, depression of immunologic reactivity actually was associated with a decrease in metastasis[31-36] or had no influence whatsoever on the growth of a local or disseminated tumor.[37] The basis for these discrepancies could have been the differences in the histology and etiology of the tumors and in the species in which they originated. In order to study the importance of host immunity to the incidence of metastasis by tumors of different antigenicities, we minimized these experimental variables. Three murine fibrosarcomas with different degrees of immunogenicities were examined for their metastatic activity in normal mice, immunosuppressed or sham-suppressed mice, and immunosuppressed mice whose T-cell immunity was reconstituted immediately before the studies.[37] A highly immunogenic fibrosarcoma grew locally and formed more pulmonary tumor colonies in immunosuppressed mice than in normal, sham-suppressed, or lymphocyte-reconstituted animals. A fibrosarcoma of intermediate immunogenicity grew locally and also formed more pulmonay metastases in immunosuppressed mice, but this increase could not be reversed by reconstitution with lymphocytes from normal mice. In sharp contrast, the third and least immunogenic fibrosarcoma produced fewer pulmonary tumor colonies in immunosuppressed mice than it did in normal, sham-suppressed, or immunoreconstituted mice. Thus, even under relatively uniform laboratory conditions, the influence of the immune system on experimental cancer metastasis varied for the three syngeneic tumors. These data demonstrate that although tumor immunogenicity is an important factor in the relationship between host immunity and tumor dissemination, no generalizations about this relationship should be drawn based on a single tumor system.[37]

III. THE BIOLOGIC HETEROGENEITY OF MALIGNANT NEOPLASMS AND ITS IMPLICATIONS FOR HOST RESISTANCE AGAINST TUMORS

There is now a large body of data to indicate that at the time of diagnosis, malignant neoplasms are heterogeneous and contain cells with diverse phenotypic characteristics such as antigenicity and immunogenicity, growth rate, protein production, karyotype, cell surface receptors, hormone receptors, response to a variety of cytotoxic drugs, and metastatic potential.[38-40] Similarly, different metastases proliferating in the same or different organs can exhibit both inter- and intralesional heterogeneity.[40-42] The inter-metastases biologic heterogeneity may be due to the clonal origin of metastases and to the fact that different metastases can originate from different progenitor cells.[43] The intralesional biologic heterogeneity observed within metastases could be due to the phenotypic instability of clonal populations (early metastasis),[44] and to the increased rate of spontaneous mutation in metastatic cells as compared with nonmetastatic cells.[45,46]

Heterogeneity in sensitivity to cytotoxic drugs exists among tumor cell subpopulations populating primary neoplasms. Cells isolated from a rat hepatocellular carcinoma,[47] a methylcholanthrene-induced murine sarcoma,[48] and a murine mammary tumor[49] have been shown to have different in vitro and in vivo sensitivities to a variety of chemotherapeutic agents. These observations are not restricted to experimental tumor systems. Various human neoplasms such as melanoma,[50] ovarian carcinoma,[51] and lymphoma[52] also have been shown to be heterogeneous for drug response. Even within the same patient, different metastases can exhibit different susceptibilities to chemotherapeutic agents.[53] The emergence of drug-resistant tumor cell variants in clinical oncology is well documented. For example, small-cell carcinoma of the lung is usually initially sensitive to chemotherapy with or without radiotherapy. In contrast, recurrences, which are a common feature of this neoplasm, are resistant to chemotherapy regardless of the magnitude of the initial response to therapy.[54,55]

Antigenic and or immunogenic heterogeneity of tumor cells also presents problems for treatment of metastasis. Analysis of several AKR murine leukemias demonstrated that these tumors were immunologically polyclonal.[56] Immunization of tumor-bearing animals with a vaccine prepared from the original tumor proved unsuccessful because only the dominant population was rejected, allowing the minor subpopulations to proliferate: the minor subpopulations in the vaccine did not offer a significant immunologic challenge for stimulation.[56] Because tumor cell variants resistant to chemotherapy or immunotherapy can proliferate unchecked following the destruction of the sensitive populations, the successful treatment of metastases will be one that can circumvent the problem of cellular diversity and that does not induce resistance.

IV. THE IN VITRO INTERACTION OF TUMOR CYTOTOXIC MONONUCLEAR PHAGOCYTES WITH TARGET CELLS

Although tumor cell populations are heterogeneous with regard to many phenotypes, they appear to be sensitive to destruction by appropriately activated (tumor cytotoxic) macrophages. Mononuclear phagocytes can be rendered tumor cytotoxic following their interaction with various natural and synthetic agents (Table 1).[4,5,57-77] Once activated, at least in vitro, macrophages acquire the ability to recognize and destroy neoplastic cells while leaving nonneoplastic cells unharmed.[78-81] The reason target cells are susceptible to destruction by activated macrophages is not understood. The susceptibility of tumor cells to destruction by tumoricidal macrophages appears to be independent of the in vivo biological behavior of the tumor cell. Melanoma variant cell lines that have a low or high metastatic potential, that have invasive or noninvasive characteristics, and that are either susceptible or resistant to lysis mediated by syngeneic T-cells or NK cells are all lysed in vitro by lymphokine-activated macrophages.[80] Similarly, several cloned cell lines that were isolated from a murine fibrosarcoma induced by UV-radiation and that vary in their degree of immunogenicity or invasive and metastatic potential in vivo[82] are all susceptible to destruction in vitro by tumoricidal macrophages. Not all investigators agree that macrophage-mediated destruction of tumor cells is independent of the metastatic potential of the cancer cell.[84,85] These reports indicate an inverse relationship between the ability of a tumor cell to form metastases and its susceptibility to destruction by activated macrophages. The susceptibility of target cells to destruction by activated macrophages has also been examined with virus-transformed cell lines in which various characteristics of the transformed phenotype are temperature-dependent.[86] These studies demonstrated that the tumor cells were lysed by macrophages regardless of whether they expressed particular cell surface protein (LETS) or Forssman antigens, displayed surface charge that permitted agglutination by low doses of plant lectins, expressed SV40-T-antigen, had a low saturation density, or exhibited density-dependent inhibition of DNA synthesis.[86] Of particular

Table 1
IMMUNOMODULATORS CAPABLE OF
ACTIVATING TUMORICIDAL PROPERTIES IN
MONONUCLEAR PHAGOCYTES

Agent	Ref.
Chronic infection of host with bacteria, protozoa, nematodes	57—59
Bacterial cell wall components	
Endotoxin, lipopolysaccharide, lipid A	60—64
Muramyl dipeptide (MDP)	65—67
dsRNA	60
Lymphokines	
Specfic macrophage arming factor (SMAF)	4, 5, 68
Macrophage Activating Factor (MAF)	61—64, 69—72
Interferon-Gamma (IFN-γ)	64, 69, 73
Aggregated IgG, immune complexes	74
C-reactive protein	75
Lysolecithin analogs	76, 77

importance in the treatment of metastasis is the observation that tumor cell variants selected for resistance to the anthracycline antibiotic Adriamycin remain fully susceptible to destruction by tumoricidal macrophages.[87]

To further understand the basis for tumor cell susceptibility to macrophage-mediated destruction, we recently attempted to select in vitro tumor cells that were resistant to lysis by activated macrophages.[88] We employed a previous technique used to select tumor cells resistant to T-lymphocytes[89] or NK cells.[9] There were seven different heterogeneous murine neoplasms and one cloned line of a fibrosarcoma cultured in vitro with syngeneic tumoricidal macrophages. Surviving tumor cells were recovered and expanded to be subsequently exposed once more to tumor cytotoxic macrophages. After six such sequential interactions, all cell lines were examined for their susceptibility to lysis mediated by activated macrophages. In all eight systems, no significant differences were detected between the parent tumor cells and cells that survived the six sequential interactions. Neither macrophage infiltration into tumors growing subcutaneously nor the experimental or spontaneous metastatic potentials of the parental tumor lines differed from the lines established by the cells surviving six cycles of macrophage-mediated lysis. Collectively, these data suggest that tumor cell destruction by activated macrophages is nonselective and does not lead to the development of resistant tumor cells or to cells with altered metastatic properties.[88]

Much of our knowledge regarding the mechanisms by which mononuclear phagocytes destroy susceptible target cells has been obtained from a variety of in vitro assays, including light microscopy,[90] inhibition of tumor growth (cytostasis),[91-93] cleared zones of tumor cell monolayers,[94,95] release of radioactive labels from target cells,[96-98] cinemicrographic analysis,[99] sequential scanning, and transmission electron microscopy.[100] Morphologic studies of the interaction of murine macrophages with susceptible target cells suggested to Hibbs[101] that a direct macrophage-target cell contact involving the transfer of lysosomal enzymes is responsible for target lysis. Evidence to support this concept was provided by the ultrastructural studies reported by Bucana et al.[100] Both investigators emphasized that macrophage binding to tumor cells followed by destabilization of the target cell membrane constitute integral steps of the cytolytic process.[100,101] Miller et al.,[102] on the other hand, examined murine peritoneal macrophages treated with perfluorochemicals and did not find evidence for the transfer of lysosomes from the activated macrophage into the target cell or alterations in the structure of adjacent macrophage-tumor membranes. Another potential mechanism of macrophage-mediated tumor cell cytotoxicity following cell-cell interaction was suggested by the findings of Kaplan et al.[103] Lewis lung carcinoma cells were found to undergo a reductive cell division in the absence of DNA synthesis following interaction with murine macrophages activated by *Corynebacterium parvum,* suggesting that this aberrant division may be related to the lethal event mediated by activated macrophages.

Not all investigators agree that direct macrophage-tumor cell contact is mandatory for destruction of target cells by macrophages. The release of soluble macrophage secretory products at contact sites with their targets has been proposed as one mechanism of indirect target cell lysis.[104-106] Other agents thought to be involved in lysis of target cells include cytotoxins released by macrophages,[107-110] the third component of complement (C3a),[111] tumor cell growth inhibitory products such as excess thymidine,[112] hydrogen peroxide,[113,114] and heat-labile neutral serine proteases.[115,116] Regardless of whether macrophages lyse tumor cells by direct binding or by the release of soluble factors, most investigators agree that, at least in vitro, activated macrophages discriminate tumorigenic from nontumorigenic cells.

V. MECHANISMS FOR THE INDUCTION AND MAINTENANCE OF TUMORICIDAL PROPERTIES IN MACROPHAGES

The cellular and molecular processes by which a nontumoricidal macrophage can become activated to the tumoricidal state are now receiving wide attention. Current concepts of this activation process suggest that a series of phenotypic alterations are acquired in a sequential fashion, culminating in the development of tumoricidal properties. The rate of appearance or loss of a specific phenotypic alteration depends on the nature and duration of activating factors.[61,117,118]

The activation of macrophages by lymphokines such as IFN-γ or macrophage-activating factor (MAF) requires that the agents bind to the macrophage surface.[119] Treatment of macrophages with reagents that alter their surface properties influences the extent to which they respond to lymphokines.[119,120] Augmentation of macrophage responses to lymphokines was observed subsequent to alteration of amino, sulphydryl, hydroxyl, or carbonyl groups on the cell surface.[121] In contrast, treatment of macrophages with various proteases or with α-L-fucose decreased their response to MAF, suggesting that fucose-containing moieties could be the receptor for MAF.[119,120] Moreover, the incubation of macrophages with liposomes containing fucoglycolipids enhanced their responses to MAF, suggesting that cell surface fucoglycolipids may be the natural receptor for MAF.[119] More recently, direct evidence has been presented for the existence of cell surface IFN-γ receptors that bind IFN-γ and thus participate in the activation of macrophage tumoricidal properties.[122]

Whether the cellular alterations in lymphokine-treated macrophages resulted directly from the binding of MAF or IFN-γ to surface receptors or whether the receptor-bound material was internalized to act at an intracellular locus was not clear. In the latter case the surface receptor would merely bind sufficient lymphokine molecules to initiate biological activity. Experimentally, these questions can be studied by assessing the ability to activate macrophages under conditions in which MAF or IFN-γ is allowed to bind to its surface receptor but not be internalized or under conditions in which the agents are introduced directly into the cell without their initial binding to surface receptors. The latter possibility has been investigated by using synthetic phospholipid vesicles (liposomes) as carrier vehicles to deliver MAF or IFN-γ directly into the intracellular matrix of the macrophages.

In studies from our laboratory, lymphokines with MAF activity were obtained from cultures of mitogen-stimulated rat lymphocytes. These lymphokines were encapsulated within liposomes of different size and lipid composition.[120,123,124] The ability of free and liposome-encapsulated MAF to render normal murine or rat macrophages cytotoxic for tumor cells in vitro was compared. Our studies revealed that normal rodent macrophages were rendered tumoricidal after incubation with liposome-encapsulated MAF and that the level of cytotoxicity exceeded that induced by free-MAF. Control cultures of macrophages incubated with liposomes alone or liposomes containing supernatants from normal unstimulated lymphocytes did not acquire tumor cytotoxic properties.

In comparing the extent of macrophage activation induced by free-MAF and by liposome-encapsulated MAF, it is important to realize that the total amount of free-MAF added to macrophages greatly exceeds the total amount of MAF encapsulated within liposomes. By using serial dilution experiments, we found that the total amount of liposome-encapsulated MAF inducing activation in macrophages was at least 4 logs lower than the volume of free-MAF that was used to induce similar activation.[120,123] The activation by liposome-encapsulated lymphokine was not due to liposome-mediated alterations in the macrophage surface that enhanced their responsiveness to MAF. We conclude this from control experiments in which macrophages incubated with liposomes containing saline and suspended in medium supplemented with MAF diluted 10,000-fold did not acquire tumoricidal properties. Further evidence that liposome-entrapped MAF activates macrophages via an intracellular mechanism comes from activation experiments in which normal macrophages were incubated with either free-MAF or liposome-encapsulated MAF in the presence of several compounds known to inhibit MAF binding to the macrophage surface. Liposome-encapsulated MAF but not free-MAF activated tumoricidal properties in macrophages concomitantly treated with α-L-fucose or p-nitrophenyl-2-0-α-L-fuco-pyranosyl-β-D-galactopyranoside. Similarly, liposome-encapsulated MAF activated macrophages that were refractory to activation by free-MAF because of treatments with pronase or α-L-fucosidase, which remove surface receptors for MAF, or with fucose-binding plant lectins (*Ulex europaeus* I and *Lotus tetragonolobus*), which compete for binding to the MAF receptor on macrophages. Moreover, populations of nontumoricidal inflammatory tissue macrophages, which were inherently unresponsive to free-MAF, could be rendered tumoricidal in vitro by incubation with liposome-encapsulated MAF.[120] Finally, liposome-encapsulated MAF activated tumoricidal properties of macrophages obtained from endotoxin-nonresponsive C3H/HeJ mice whereas free-MAF did not.[125] Collectively, then, our studies indicate that the activation of macrophages by MAF does not require binding of the lymphokine to the macrophage surface receptors. These initial investigations on the activation of tumoricidal properties in rodent macrophages by liposome-encapsulated MAF have now been expanded to a human system with equivalent results: the activation of normal, noncytotoxic human blood monocytes by human MAF does not require binding of the lymphokine to putative monocyte surface receptors.[126]

Mononuclear phagocytes can also be rendered tumoricidal by a variety of microorganisms and their structural components (Table 1). One such component of bacterial cell wall, N-acetylmuramyl-L-alanyl-D-isoglutamine (muramyl dipeptide, MDP) has been shown to be the minimal active unit with immune-potentiating activity that can replace *Mycobacterium* in complete Freund's adjuvant. The mechanism by which MDP activates monocyte/macrophage function has been investigated in both rodent[129] and human[130] systems with radiolabeled glycopeptides. Collectively, the results indicate the absence of cell surface MDP receptors and suggest that the activation of tumoricidal properties in mononuclear phagocytes by muramyl peptides occurs as the result of an intracytoplasmic event following pinocytosis of the glycopeptide.[129,130]

The absence of cell surface receptors for MDP on mononuclear phagocytes is not surprising. In contrast to the activation of macrophages by lymphokines, naturally occurring MDP is liberated following the phagocytosis of bacteria and the breakdown of bacterial cell walls within the macrophage cytoplasm.[125,131] In nature, therefore, muramyl dipeptides are presented to the macrophage through an intracellular pathway. In this regard, several laboratories have documented this ability of liposome-encapsulated MDP (and various analogs) to activate tumoricidal properties in both rodent[67,125,132-135] and human[136-139] macrophages following phagocytosis of the phospholipid vesicle.

The activation of tumor cytotoxic properties in macrophages by lymphokines or bacterial components need not occur independently of each other. A lymphokine such as IFN-γ[140-142] or MAF[143-145] can prime macrophages to respond to a second signal such as endotoxins[143,144,146] or MDP.[144,145] Recent studies from our laboratory have concentrated on the synergistic activation of tumoricidal properties in macrophages by recombinant IFN- and MDP.[147-149] We found that human blood monocytes and murine peritoneal exudate macrophages were activated by the combination of subthreshold amounts of MDP and recombinant IFN-γ to become tumoricidal against their human or murine tumorigenic target cells.[147-149] The activation of human monocytes or murine macrophages by free-IFN-γ and MDP was species specific: human IFN-γ did not activate murine macrophages; and murine IFN-γ did not activate cytotoxic properties in human monocytes. In both species, the activation of tumoricidal properties in macrophages by IFN-γ occurred as a consequence of intracellular interaction. We base this conclusion on data showing that, whereas free IFN-γ and MDP did not activate macrophages pretreated with pronase, liposome-encapsulated IFN-γ and MDP did.[149] Moreover, the encapsulation of either murine or human IFN-γ with MDP within the same liposome preparation produced synergistic activation of cytotoxic properties in both mouse macrophages and human monocytes without apparent species specificity.[149] These data suggest that, at least functionally, IFN-γ consists of two separate moieties. One part may be responsible for binding to the macrophage surface to facilitate the internalization of part of or the whole molecule. This moiety of the IFN-γ molecule may be responsible for the intracellular activation of macrophages to the tumoricidal state, which is not species specific.

Once macrophages have undergone the sequence of phenotypic alterations resulting in activation, they rapidly lose their cytolytic activity when isolated in vitro. Prostaglandins of the E series (PGE) may mediate such loss, a possibility suggested by the findings that cyclooxgenase inhibitors such as indomethacin prevent both the synthesis of PGE and the loss of cytolytic activity by lymphokine-activated macrophages.[150,151] This may not be a universal finding, since in another study, indomethacin had either no effect or an inhibitory effect on macrophage activation.[152] Another recent report has implicated neuropeptide levels as an important determinant in macrophage tumoricidal activity.[153]

It is apparent that the results of an in vitro assay that measures macrophage-mediated cytotoxicity could differ vastly according to the conditions of the experiment. For a detailed discussion of these experimental variables, the reader is referred to a recent editorial.[154] The lack of standardization of many experimental conditions could indeed be responsible for many conflicting reports regarding activation of tumoricidal properties in macrophages and their in vitro interaction with tumor cell populations.

VI. THE INVOLVEMENT OF THE MONONUCLEAR PHAGOCYTE SYSTEM IN THE INITIATION AND PROGRESSION OF CANCER

The macrophage participates in a number of host homeostatic mechanisms that include the clearance and catabolism of red blood cells and debris,[155] the controlled recycling of iron stores,[156] and the metabolism of lipids.[157] When host homeostatic mechanisms are stressed, the mononuclear phagocyte system can participate in complex interactions that involve cellular and humoral aspects of the inflammatory and immunologic responses.[158-161] In this regard, the macrophage is recognized as an important component of the host defense system against viral, bacterial, fungal, and parasitic infections.[158,159] Mononuclear phagocytes also affect the pathogenesis and development of neoplasms.[162-163]

Macrophages may play a prominent role in the detection and destruction of neoplastic cells by the host immune surveillance system.[94,164] An early investigation using tumor systems in rabbits produced evidence that the incidence of uterine cancer, dependent on age and strain, was parallel to the natural resistance to infection by tuberculosis (the most resistant strain having the lowest incidence of cancer).[165] In addition, the resistance of the rabbits to tuberculosis was directly related to the bactericidal capacity of their mononuclear phagocyte system.[165] These studies suggested a correlation between the activity of the phagocytes and the observed resistance to neoplasia. Subsequent studies supported this concept. Mice infected with the intracellular protozoa *Toxoplasma gondii* were more resistant to viral induction of neoplasms and to tumors resulting from the transplantation of syngeneic tumor cells.[166] The macrophages harvested from the protozoa-infected mice were cytotoxic in vitro to the transplanted tumor cells.[166] The importance of macrophages in carcinogenesis was revealed by studies designed to determine whether treatment of mice with either a macrophage stimulant (pyran copolymer) or macrophage toxins (trypan blue or silica) would influence the latency or incidence of skin carcinogenesis induced by UV-radiation. Treatment of mice with pyran copolymer lengthened the latent period of tumor development and reduced the incidence and number of the skin tumors that resulted from suboptimal exposures to UV-radiation.[167] Conversely, treatment of mice with macrophage toxins shortened the latent period for induction of skin cancer by UV-radiation.[167] Similarly, in transplantable tumor systems, the impairment of macrophage function by agents such as carrageenan or silica was found to be associated with an increase in the incidence of spontaneous[168,169] and experimental metastases.[170] There are also several reports regarding the efficacy of macrophages in the inhibition of metastasis. In an adoptive transfer study, i.v. injections of syngeneic murine macrophages that had been rendered tumoricidal by in vivo or in vitro manipulation reduced the incidence of experimental metastases of the B16 melanoma.[171] Similarly, activated macrophages have been shown to eradicate metastases in two other murine tumor systems,[172,173] and to inhibit the growth of tumors at primary sites.[174]

Progressively growing tumors can induce several alterations in macrophage function, such as enhanced carbon clearance in vivo,[175,176] increased expression of monocyte Fc receptors,[177,178] suppressed migration of macrophages into the peritoneal cavity or the site of subcutaneously growing tumors, and suppressed chemotactic response of macrophages in these sites.[179-184] In this context, we investigated whether the presence of progressively growing metastases in lung parenchyma of rats influenced the number and function of lung macrophages.[185] The presence of pulmonary metastases (produced by a syngeneic mammary adenocarcinoma) did not result in a decrease in the number of lung macrophages, and the macrophages harvested from rats with metastases were functionally intact.[185] Furthermore, the macrophages harvested from rats with metastases could be rendered cytotoxic to syngeneic tumor cells in response to activation stimuli administered in vitro or in vivo.[185] Such findings suggest that the presence of a large number of tumor cells in organ parenchyma need not interfere with the function of macrophages in that organ.

Although the presence of macrophages at the periphery of and within neoplasms is well recognized, their functional activity is unclear. Differences in the cytotoxic activity of macrophages isolated from nonmetastasizing and metastasizing tumors have been reported.[186] Mononuclear phagocytes isolated from a nonmetastatic sarcoma demonstrated cytotoxicity in vitro.[186] In contrast, intratumoral macrophages of a weakly immunogenic, metastasizing tumor were not demonstrably cytotoxic. Similar data have been reported for progressing and regressing murine sarcomas.[187] These data are not universal. Other investigators have observed the converse to be true; i.e. intratumoral macrophages of metastasizing tumors and to a lesser extent nonmetastasizing tumors are indeed cytotoxic.[188] Moreover, macrophage-mediated cytotoxicity in vitro could not always be correlated with the in vivo behavior of the tumor from which the macrophages were isolated.[189]

Preliminary studies found that the macrophage content of six carcinogen-induced rat fibrosarcomas correlated directly with their immunogenicity and inversely with their metastatic potential, suggesting that some tumors are nonmetastatic because they contain many macrophages.[190,191] Once again, such observations could not be extended to other tumor systems. We examined the macrophage content of 16 different rodent tumors and did not find a correlation between the extent of macrophage infiltration into neoplasms and the metastatic behavior of the tumors.[192] Similar results have now been reported for several other tumor systems.[193,194] Interestingly, in one of these reports differences between metastatic and nonmetastatic tumors were seen in the density and size of macrophages, macrophage ectoenzyme concentrations, and macrophage-associated PGE levels.[194]

Several factors influence the extent of macrophage infiltration into tumors. One factor, tumor cell immunogenicity, did not correlate with macrophage content in our study.[192] This observation is in agreement with studies by others, who examined the macrophage content of 33 different methylcholanthrene-induced murine fibrosarcomas and rhabdomyosarcomas and concluded that there was no relationship between macrophage content and the immunogenicity of the tumors.[195,196] The factors influencing macrophage infiltration into tumors are poorly understood, but both immune and nonimmune factors are clearly involved.[195] In fact, many tumors appear to be nonimmunogenic under conditions of progressive growth, and in these tumors, macrophage infiltration may depend more on nonimmunologic factors such as inflammation and necrosis.[197]

Whether tumors regress or progress can be determined by the degree to which tumoricidal activity of macrophages is generated *in situ,* rather than by the number of macrophages within the tumor.[187] This finding could explain why progressively growing spontaneous metastases often contain as many or more macrophages than the parent tumor.[198] Recently, two independent studies reported that the macrophage content of pooled metastases were similar to that of primary tumors[193] and that the metastases did not consist of cells resistant to macrophage-mediated lysis.[199]

Clearly, the role of the mononuclear phagocyte system in metastasis varies among different tumors and need not correlate with tumor cell immunogenicity or metastatic properties. In some tumors, numerous infiltrating macrophages can inhibit metastasis, but the absence of macrophage infiltration of a benign neoplasm will not lead to metastasis. Thus, neoplasms with low macrophage content may or may not be metastatic, as demonstrated by studies in which nonmetastatic clones isolated from a highly metastatic neoplasm also exhibited low macrophage content when growing subcutaneously.[198]

VII. THE IN VIVO ACTIVATION OF THE MONONUCLEAR PHAGOCYTE SYSTEM FOR TREATMENT OF METASTASES

The i.v. injection of syngeneic, macrophages that were nonspecifically activated in vitro into mice with metastatic lesions has been shown to inhibit tumor growth both at the primary site[174] and in metastases.[171-173] These findings suggested that the i.v. administration of tumor cytotoxic macrophages might augment host resistance to disseminated cancer. The clinical feasibility of this approach, however, suffers from two shortcomings: it requires a large number of autologous or histocompatible macrophages for transfusion, and most intravenously injected macrophages arrest in the pulmonary microvasculature and do not reach other visceral organs. A more promising approach, therefore, has been the development of a method to activate host mononuclear phagocytes *in situ.*

One of the major pathways for the activation of macrophages in vivo involves their direct interaction with microorganisms and their structural components. Because such materials are often associated with undesirable side effects, such as delayed type hypersensitivity and granuloma formation,[200] it is preferable to use synthetic compounds that are less toxic yet capable of inducing the in vivo activation of macrophages. One such synthetic agent, MDP (and various analogs), profoundly influences many macrophage functions including cytotoxic activity in vitro.[201,202] Following parenteral administration, however, this compound is rapidly cleared (1 to 2 hr) from the body by the kidneys.[203,204] This short half-life limits the therapeutic potential of MDP.

A second major pathway for macrophage activation in vivo results from the action of lymphokines (MAF and IFN-γ) released from sensitized lymphocytes. Therapeutic use of soluble MAF or soluble IFN-γ has been hindered in the past by the lack of purified preparations of these mediators. Efforts to activate the tumoricidal properties of macrophages in vivo by systemic injection of crude lymphokine preparations have proved unsuccessful. Injection of soluble lymphokines into skin[205] or skin tumors[206,207] provoked local inflammatory reactions and histologic changes suggestive of macrophage activation that resulted in the regression of small cutaneous tumors. Systemic activation of macrophages by free-lymphokines, however, has not been achieved. There are several reasons for this failure:

1. Lymphokines injected into venous circulation have a short half-life,[208] probably because they bind with plasma proteins.[209]
2. Only a small fraction of the mononuclear phagocyte system may be capable of responding to MAF.
3. Macrophages can be activated by lymphokines only within a relatively short period following their emigration into tissues from the circulation.[209]
4. The tumoricidal properties of macrophages are short-lived (2 to 3 days), and macrophages are refractory to reactivation by soluble lymphokines.[209]

Studies from our laboratory[67,120,123-126,132-134,144,145] and subsequently by others[75,135-137] have shown that the phagocytic uptake by macrophages of liposomes containing macrophage-activating agents produces highly efficient activation of rodent and human macrophages in vitro. These findings raised the possibility that agents encapsulated within liposomes could be similarly efficient in activating macrophages in vivo. An attractive feature of liposomes as carriers for delivering agents to macrophages *in situ* is that most of the liposomes injected intravenously are taken up by phagocytic cells of the reticuloendothelial system. This passive targeting of liposomes offers a means of enhancing uptake of agents that stimulate macrophage activity.[210,211] Moreover, liposomes prepared from natural phospholipids are nonimmunogenic, and thus they offer a way to avoid eliciting the allergic reactions commonly associated with the systemic administration of immune adjuvants.[212]

To test this possibility, mice with spontaneous pulmonary and lymph node metastases were injected intravenously with MAF encapsulated within multilamellar liposomes composed of phosphatidylcholine and phosphatidylserine. This type of liposome was chosen for several reasons. First, studies of body distribution of liposomes of different size and phospholipid composition demonstrated that these negatively charged liposomes localize and are retained in the lungs (in addition to organs rich with reticuloendothelial cell activity).[213] Second, toxicity studies in which these liposomes containing MAF were injected intravenously into mice or beagle dogs revealed no adverse reactions in recipient animals even after repeated injections.[214] Finally, another study has shown that i.v. injection of these liposomes activates murine or rat lung macrophages to become tumoricidal.[215]

In the initial studies, multiple i.v. injections of liposome-encapsulated MAF, but not soluble MAF or control liposome preparations, led to the eradication of spontaneous visceral metastases in C57BL/6 mice subsequent to surgical excision of syngeneic melanoma growing subcutaneously.[216] To initiate local tumors, each mouse was given an intrafootpad injection of viable B16-BL6 melanoma cells. When the primary tumor reached a size of 1.0 to 1.2 cm in diameter (4 weeks of growth), the tumor-bearing leg, including the draining popliteal lymph node, was amputated. Treatment of mice began 3 days after leg amputation and consisted of an i.v. injection of 2.5 μmol liposomes (phosphatidylcholine and phosphatidylserine admixed at a 7:3 mole ratio) containing 6.25 $\mu\ell$ of MAF. Mice were treated twice weekly for 4 weeks (total of 8 i.v. injections). The B16-BL6 tumor routinely metastasizes to the lungs and lymph nodes in about 90% of untreated mice, and at the start of therapy, the metastatic tumor burden in the lungs and lymph nodes may have exceeded a total body burden of 10^7 cells. Nonetheless, 70% of mice treated with liposome-encapsulated MAF survived at least 200 days. The median life span of mice implanted with ten viable B16 cells admixed with 10^6 dead cells is 40 to 50 days.[217] For this reason, it is most likely that the tumor burden was reduced to fewer than ten viable cells in the successfully treated mice. Thus, multiple i.v. injections of liposome-encapsulated MAF brought about the complete regression of established pulmonary and lymph node metastases.

In the above studies, the use of crude lymphokine preparations with multiple immune-potentiating activities including MAF complicated delineation of the mechanism involved during the successful treatment of metastases. To investigate this issue, and to further examine the therapeutic implications of liposomes containing macrophage-activating agents in cancer metastases, we used synthetic MDP.[132] The principal target cell for immune modulation by MDP is believed to be the macrophage.[201,202] Recent studies from our laboratory have shown that MDP encapsulated within liposomes can render macrophages tumoricidal in vitro much more efficiently than free, unencapsulated MDP.[67,133] In contrast to free-MDP, liposome-encapsulated MDP requires less time (2 hr) to activate macrophages, and maximum cytolytic capacity is achieved after an 8-hr incubation.[67] Furthermore, the total amount of liposome-encapsulated MDP that is delivered to macrophages is at least 4000 times lower than the total amount of free-MDP necessary to render macrophages tumoricidal.[67,133] Finally, after the initial activation period, liposome-encapsulated MDP can prolong the duration of tumoricidal properties in macrophages.[133]

We have recently studied the organ distribution and retention of free and liposome-encapsulated MDP (^{3}H-labeled) following i.v. administration into mice.[218] In agreement with previous studies,[203,204] we found that by 2 hr after its administration, more than 90% of free-MDP was cleared from the body and excreted in the urine. However, the excretion rate of liposome-encapsulated MDP was 3 to 6%/hr and the percentage of the total dose of liposome-encapsulated MDP that localized in the liver, spleen, and lung was increased 10- to 30-fold over that of free-MDP. Moreover, liposome encapsulation delayed the onset of MDP metabolite production.[218] In this regard, the injection of MDP in saline did not render alveolar macrophages of mice tumoricidal, whereas injection of MDP encapsulated in liposomes did activate the alveolar macrophages to become tumoricidal against B16-BL6 melanoma cells, and the systemic activation of macrophages by liposome-encapsulated MDP can be maintained by repeated injections.[132,133,219] Finally, in the melanoma therapy model the i.v. injection of liposome-encapsulated MDP, but not free-MDP, destroyed established pulmonary and lymph node metastases.[132]

The mechanisms responsible for the regression of established metastases after the systemic administration of liposomes containing MDP or MAF probably involved the activation of macrophages to become tumoricidal. Several lines of evidence tend to support this conclusion. First, lung macrophages are not activated by macrophage-activating agents encapsulated within liposomes that are not retained in the lung.[220] Second, the pretreatment of tumor-bearing animals with agents that are toxic for macrophages (silica, carrageenan, hyperchlorinated drinking water) before systemic therapy with liposome-encapsulated MDP or MAF abrogates the response to liposome therapy, and such animals rapidly die of metastatic disease.[220] Third, the possible involvement of T-lymphocytes as effector cells is excluded by the finding that systemic activation of macrophages by liposome-encapsulated MDP can be accomplished in athymic nude mice and in adult thymectomized or X-irradiated mice.[221] Fourth, i.v. injections of macrophages activated in vitro by incubation with liposome-encapsulated MDP produces a reduction in metastatic burden comparable to that achieved by systemic administration of liposome-encapsulated activators.[220] Finally, direct evidence that the regression of established metastases after treatment of tumor-bearing mice with liposome-encapsulated activators was associated with tumoricidal macrophages comes from morphological and functional analysis of macrophages isolated from pulmonary metastases.[222] Immunofluorescence and electron microscopic analyses revealed that 24 hr after the tumor-bearing mice were given i.v. injections of liposomes, 15% of the alveolar macrophages and 5% of the metastasis-associated macrophages contained phagocytosed liposomes. However, only macrophages isolated from lungs or metastases of mice given injections of liposomes containing activators (treatment success), but not macrophages from mice treated with empty liposomes (treatment failure), were tumoricidal against the target cells in vitro.

VIII. POTENTIATION OF MACROPHAGE ACTIVATION FOR TREATMENT OF CANCER METASTASES WITH LIPOSOME-ENCAPSULATED AGENTS

Since the original demonstration that the activation of tumoricidal properties in mononuclear phagocytes by liposome-encapsulated lymphokines or MDP is associated with eradication of cancer metastasis, several laboratories began to investigate novel compounds in similar and different tumor models (Table 2). Such compounds include other lymphokine preparations or C-reactive protein encapsulated in liposomes for treatment of pulmonary or liver metastases arising from the T241 murine fibrosarcoma and MCA-38 colon carcinoma, respectively,[223-225] and liposome-entrapped lipophilic derivatives of MDP for macrophage activation and therapy of B16 lung metastases.[135,226,227]

Our studies have clearly shown that MDP encapsulated within liposomes renders macrophages tumoricidal much more effectively than does unencapsulated MDP.[67,132,133,219,221] Moreover, once macrophages have phagocytosed liposomes con-

Table 2

THERAPY OF SPONTANEOUS AND EXPERIMENTAL METASTASES WITH LIPOSOME-ENCAPSULATED MACROPHAGE ACTIVATING AGENTS

Tumor system	Macrophage activator	Dose and regimen agent	Results	Ref.
B16-BL-6 implanted s.c. into C57BL/6 mice. Spontaneous metastases occur in lung and lymph nodes	Lymphokine (MAF)	2.5 μmol phospholipid (MLV, PC/PS 7:3) containing 6.25 $\mu\ell$ MAF, multiple doses beginning day 3 after tumor amputation	Decrease in pulmonary nodules and increase in long-term survivors	216
	MDP	2.5 μmol phospholipid (MLV, PC/PS 7:3) containing 6.25 μg MDP, multiple doses beginning day 3 after tumor amputation	Decrease in pulmonary nodules and increase in long-term survivors	132
	MTP-PE	2.5 μmol phospholipid (MLV, PC/PS 7:3) containing 10 μg MTP-PE, multiple doses beginning day 7 after tumor amputation	Decrease in pulmonary nodules and increase in long-term survivors	226
	Lymphokine (MAF) + MDP	2.5 μmol phospholipid (MLV, PC/PS 7:3) containing 0.31 $\mu\ell$ MAF and 0.3 μg MDP, multiple doses beginning day 7 after tumor amputation	Decrease in pulmonary nodules and increase in long-term survivors	145
T241 fibrosarcoma injected s.c. into C57BL/6 mice. Spontaneous lung metastases	Lymphokine (MAF)	2.5 μmol phospholipid (MLV, PC/PS 1:1) containing 6.25 $\mu\ell$ MAF, multiple doses beginning day 3 after tumor amputation	Decrease in pulmonary nodules and increase in long-term survivors	223
	CRP	2.5 μmol phospholipid (MLV, PC/PS 1:1) containing 0.7 μg CRP, multiple doses beginning day 3 after tumor implantation	Decrease in pulmonary nodules and increase in long-term survivors	224
MCA-38 orthotopic transplantation into the cecum of C57BL/6 mice. Liver metastases	CRP or Lymphokine (MAF)	4 μmol phospholipid (MLV, PC/PS 1:1) containing 10 $\mu\ell$ MAF or 1.1 μg CRP, multiple doses beginning day 2 after tumor inoculation	Decrease in liver nodules and increase in long-term survivors	225
B16 melanoma injected i.v. into C57BL/6 mice. Lung metastases	6-O-S[Abu]MDP	2 μmol phospholipid (MLV, DOPC/DOPG 7:3) containing 60 μg 6-O-S[Abu]MDP, multiple doses beginning day 3 after tumor inoculation	Decrease in lung nodules	227

B16 melanoma injected i.v. into C67BL/6 mice	MDP-GDP	0.5 μmol phospholipid (MLV, DSPC/PS 7:3) containing 10 μg MDP-GDP, multiple doses beginning day 3 after tumor inoculation	Decrease in lung nodules	135
Nonimmunogenic fibrosarcoma injected i.v. into C3Hf/Kam mice. Lung metastases	6-O-S[Abu]MDP	2 μmol phospholipid (MLV, DMPC/DMPG 7:3) containing 32-64 μg 6-O-S[Abu]MDP, multiple doses beginning day 3 after tumor inoculation	Decrease in lung nodules	227
Fibrosarcoma injected i.v. into C3Hf/Kam mice. Lung metastases	6-O-S[Abu]MDP	2 μmol phospholipid (MLV, DMPC, DMPG 7:3) containing 32-64 μg 6-O-S[Abu]MDP, multiple doses beginning day 3 after tumor inoculation	Decrease in lung nodules	227

taining MDP, they remain cytotoxic for 2 to 3 days.[132,133,219] Recent studies have suggested that lipophilic derivatives of MDP, in which acyl chains are attached to the molecule, enhance the effectiveness of MDP for priming peritoneal macrophages to release superoxide anion.[228] Because low molecular solutes such as hydrophilic MDP can leak out of liposomes, we examined the possibility of whether a lipophilic derivative of MDP, N-acetylmuramyl-L-alanyl-D-isoglutamyl-L-alanyl-2(1′,2′-dipalmitoyl-sn-glycero-3′ phosphoryl)-ethylamide (MTP-PE) inserted in the phospholipid bilayers of liposomes could be retained more efficiently within macrophages, thereby promoting longer periods of tumoricidal activity.[229]

The superiority of liposomes containing the lipophilic MTP-PE over liposomes containing water-soluble MDP for in vitro or in vivo activation of macrophages was demonstrated in several ways.[229] First, the i.v. injection of liposomes containing a dose of MTP-PE equal to MDP led to higher levels of alveolar macrophage-mediated cytotoxicity. Second, alveolar macrophages harvested from mice given i.v. injection of liposomes containing MTP-PE maintained their tumoricidal activity for a longer period (5 days) than macrophages harvested from mice inoculated with liposome-encapsulated MDP (3 days). Similar results were obtained from experiments dealing with macrophage activation in vitro.

It has been suggested that once macrophages phagocytose liposomes containing MDP, the liposomes function as a slow-release depot from which encapsulated material is released over a sustained period of time.[67,133] The extent of release and the possible equilibration of MDP with the extracellular medium are determined by the integrity of liposome membranes. However, MTP-PE, which is only slightly soluble in water, would remain active for longer periods, until it is degraded. Since liposomes can be seen inside macrophages for several days after phagocytosis,[230] the degradation of MTP-PE incorporated into the liposome phospholipid bilayer is apparently relatively slow and inefficient.

The increased efficacy of lipophilic MTP-PE over MDP for the in vivo activation of macrophages was also observed for therapy of spontaneous pulmonary and lymph node metastases.[226] In these experiments, the survival of tumor-bearing mice that received liposome-entrapped MTP-PE was significantly increased and obtained with fewer treatments compared with those animals given injections of liposome-encapsulated MDP. Similar results have been reported for two other lipophilic derivatives of MDP, 6-O-stearoyl-N-acetylmuramyl-L-α-aminobutyryl-D-isoglutamine (6-O-S[Abu] MDP) and α(N-acetylmuramyl-L-alanyl-D-isoglutaminyl), β, γ-dipalmitoyl-sn-glycerol (MDP-GDP).[135]

Liposomes could also deliver more than one agent to macrophages and previous studies from our laboratory have demonstrated that MAF and MDP entrapped within the same liposome preparation can act synergistically to render rat alveolar macrophages tumoricidal in vitro.[144] Moreover, the multiple systemic administration of liposomes containing both MAF and MDP into tumor-bearing mice produced synergistic activation of macrophages, which in turn were responsible for eradication of established lymph node and lung metastases.[145] In this study, it should be noted that we deliberately postponed the start of treatment to examine the hypotheses that MDP and MAF packaged within the same MLV would synergistically activate macrophages *in situ*. Specifically, i.v. injections of MLV containing an optimal dose of MAF or MDP led to regression of metastases in at least one third of the mice treated. MLV containing diluted MAF or diluted MDP had no such effects. On the other hand, the i.v. injections of MLV containing subthreshold amounts of both MAF and MDP significantly increased in long-term survival of mice (50%, $p = 0.0007$).[145]

IX. SUMMARY

The emergence of metastases resistant to conventional therapy could be the major reason for the failure to cure cancer metastasis. Tumors are heterogeneous with regard to many characteristics, including metastatic potential, and the proliferation of a minor subpopulation of cells within the primary tumor could cause treatment-resistant metastases to emerge; therefore, the successful approach to destruction of metastases will be one that circumvents tumor cell heterogeneity and does not induce resistance.

At least in vitro, appropriately activated macrophages appear able to recognize and destroy neoplastic cells regardless of other biologic phenotypes, and target cells do not appear to develop resistance to macrophage-mediated cytotoxicity. A significant effort is now under way in many laboratories to develop effective agents that will stimulate the antitumor activities of macrophages. Liposomes offer a most suitable carrier system for delivering agents to macrophages in vivo. When injected intravenously, the majority of liposomes are taken by phagocytic reticuloendothelial cells in the liver and spleen and by circulating monocytes. This provides a highly effective mechanism for targeting of liposome-encapsulated materials to macrophages. We have exploited this mechanism to deliver lymphokines and synthetic MDP to macrophages *in situ*. I.V. administration of lymphokines or MDP encapsulated in multilamellar liposomes activates macrophages in vivo and augments host resistance to metastases. No beneficial effects are obtained with the same materials administered in unencapsulated form.

Not all mice treated with i.v. injections of liposomes containing immunomodulators survived. However, the metastases of treatment-failure animals were not populated by macrophage-resistant tumor cells, indicating that macrophage activation could overcome the fundamental problem of phenotypic heterogeneity among tumor cells.[231]

The optimal conditions for systemic therapy with liposome-encapsulated immunomodulators and the efficacy of this modality alone and in combination in treating large metastatic tumor burdens are now being defined. As with many other antitumor therapies, optimal application of macrophage treatment for metastasis requires combination with other antitumor agents. Indeed, the most likely role for tumoricidal macrophages is in the destruction of micrometastases or the few tumor cells that remain after treatment with conventional adjuvant therapies such as chemotherapy.

REFERENCES

1. Fidler, I. J., Gersten, D. M., and Hart, I. R., The biology of cancer invasion and metastasis, *Adv. Cancer Res.*, 28, 149, 1978a.
2. Sugarbaker, E. V., Cancer metastasis: a product of tumor-host interactions, *Curr. Probl. Cancer*, 7, 3, 1979.
3. Poste, G. and Fidler, I. J., The pathogenesis of cancer metastasis, *Nature (London)*, 283, 139, 1979.
4. Evans, R. and Alexander, P., Rendering macrophages specifically cytotoxic by a factor released from immune lymphoid cells, *Transplantation*, 12, 227, 1971.
5. Evans, R., Grant, C. K., Cox, H., Steele, K., and Alexander, P., Thymus-derived lymphocytes produce an immunologically specific macrophage-arming factor, *J. Exp. Med.*, 136, 1318, 1972.
6. Henney, C., On the mechanism of T-cell mediated cytolysis, *Transplant. Rev.*, 17, 37, 1973.
7. Hellstrom, K. E. and Hellstrom, I., Lymphocyte-mediated cytotoxicity and blocking serum activity to tumor antigens, *Adv. Immunol.*, 18, 209, 1974.
8. Herberman, R. B. and Holden, H. T., Natural cell-mediated immunity, *Adv. Cancer Res.*, 27, 305, 1978.
9. Hanna, N. and Fidler, I. J., Role of natural killer cells in the destruction of circulating tumor emboli, *J. Natl. Cancer Inst.*, 65, 801, 1980.

10. Stutman, O., Paige, C. J., and Figarella, E. F., Natural cytotoxic cells against solid tumors in mice. I. Strain and age distribution and target cell susceptibility, *J. Immunol.*, 121, 1819, 1978.

11. Paige, C. J., Figarella, E. F., Cuttito, M. J., Cahan, A., and Stutman, O., Natural cytotoxic cells against solid tumors in mice. II. Some characteristics of the effector cells against solid tumors in mice, *J. Immunol.*, 121, 1827, 1978.

12. Nathan, C. F. and Klebanoff, S. J. Augmentation of spontaneous macrophage-mediated cytolysis by eosinophil peroxidase, *J. Exp. Med.*, 155, 1291, 1982.

13. Gorer, P. and Amos, D. B., Passive immunity of mice againt C57BL leukosis EL 4 by means of 180 immune serum, *Cancer Res.*, 16, 338, 1956.

14. Gorer, P. A. and O'Gorman, P., The cytotoxic activity of isoantibodies in mice, *Transplant. Bull.*, 3, 142, 1956.

15. Irie, K., Irie, R. F., and Morton, D. L., Evidence of in vivo reaction of antibody and complement to surface antigens of human cancer cells, *Science*, 186, 454, 1974.

16. Bodurtha, A. J., Chee, D. O., Laucius, J. F., Mastrangelo, M. J., and Prehn, R. T., Clinical and immunological significance of human melanoma cytotoxic antibody, *Cancer Res.*, 35, 189, 1975.

17. Carswell, E. A., Old, L. J., Kassel, R. L., Green, S., Fiore, N., and Williams, B., An endotoxin-induced serum factor that causes necrosis of tumors, *Proc. Natl. Acad. Sci. U.S.A.*, 72, 3666, 1975.

18. Green, S., Dobrjansky, A., Chiasso, M. A., Carswell, E., Schwartz, M. K., and Old, L. J., *Corynebacterium parvum* as the priming agent in the production of tumor necrosis factor in the mouse, *J. Natl. Cancer Inst.*, 59, 1519, 1977.

19. Kolb, W. P. and Granger, G. A., Lymphocyte in vitro cytotoxicity: characterization of mouse lymphotoxin, *Cell. Immunol.*, 1, 122, 1970.

20. Vailleur, D., Donner, M., Vailleur, J., and Burg, C., Release of lymphotoxins by spleen cells sensitized against mouse tumor associated antigens, *Cell. Immunol.*, 6, 466, 1973.

21. Heppner, G. and Miller, B. E., Biological variability of mouse mammary neoplasms, in *Design of Models for Testing Cancer Therapeutic Agents,* Fidler, I. J. and White, R. J., Eds., Van Nostrand, New York, 1981, 37.

22. Kim, U., Metastasizing mammary carcinomas in rats: induction and study of their immunogenicity, *Science*, 167, 72, 1970.

23. Fidler, I. J., Gersten, D. M., and Riggs, C. W., Relationship of host immune status to tumor cell arrest, distribution, and survival in experimental metastasis, *Cancer*, 40, 46, 1977.

24. Wexler, H., Chretien, P. B., Ketcham, A. S., and Sindelar, W. F., Induction of pulmonary metastasis in both immune and nonimmune mice: effect of the removal of a transplanted primary tumor, *Cancer*, 36, 2042, 1975.

25. Milas, L., Hunter, N., Mason, K., and Withers, H. R., Immunological resistance to pulmonary metastases in C3Hf/Bu mice bearing syngeneic fibrosarcoma of different sizes, *Cancer Res.*, 34, 61, 1974.

26. Gershon, R. K., Carter, R. L., and Kondo, K., On concomitant immunity in tumour-bearing hamsters, *Nature (London)*, 213, 674, 1967.

27. Deodhar, S. D. and Crile, G., Jr., Enhancement of metastases by antilymphocyte serum in allogeneic murine tumor system, *Cancer Res.*, 29, 776, 1969.

28. Gershon, R. K. and Carter, R. L., Facilitation of metastatic growth by antilymphocyte serum, *Nature (London)*, 226, 368, 1970.

29. Vaage, J., Chen, K., and Merrick, S., Effect of immune status on the development of artificially induced metastases in different anatomical locations, *Cancer Res.*, 31, 496, 1971.

30. Vaage, J., Humoral and cellular immune factors in the systemic control of artificially induced metastases in C3Hf mice, *Cancer Res.*, 33, 1957, 1973.

31. Fisher, E. R., Role of thymus in skin and tumor transplantation in the rat, *Lab. Invest.*, 14, 546, 1965.

32. Fidler, I. J., Immune stimulation-inhibition of experimental cancer metastasis, *Cancer Res.*, 34, 491, 1974A.

33. Umiel, T. and Trainin, N., Immunological enhancement of tumor growth by syngeneic thymus-derived lymphocytes, *Transplantation*, 18, 244, 1974.

34. Hewitt, H. B., Blake, E. R., and Walder, A. S., A critique of the evidence for active host defense against cancer, based on personal studies of 27 murine tumours of spontaneous origin, *Br. J. Cancer*, 33, 241, 1976.

35. Vaage, J., A survey of the growth characteristics of, and host reactions to, one hundred C3H/He mammary carcinomas, *Cancer Res.*, 38, 331, 1978.

36. Hager, C., Miller, F. R., and Heppner, G. H., Influence of serial transplantation on the immunological-clinical correlates of BALB/cf C3H mouse mammary tumors, *Cancer Res.*, 38, 2492, 1978.

37. Fidler, I. J., Gertsen, D. M., and Kripke, M. L., Influence of immune status on the metastasis of three murine fibrosarcomas of different immunogenicities, *Cancer Res.*, 39, 3816, 1979b.

38. Fidler, I. J., Tumor heterogeneity and the biology of cancer invasion and metastasis, *Cancer Res.,* 37, 2481, 1978a.
39. Fidler, I. J. and Hart, I. R., The origin of metastatic heterogeneity in tumors, *Eur. J. Cancer,* 17, 487, 1981.
40. Hart, I. R. and Fidler, I. J., The implications of tumor heterogeneity for studies on the biology and therapy of cancer metastasis, *Biochim. Biophys. Acta,* 651, 37, 1981.
41. Calabresi, P., Dexter, D. L., and Heppner, G. H., Clinical and pharmacological implications of cancer cell differentiation and heterogeneity, *Biochem. Pharmacol.,* 28, 1933, 1979.
42. Fidler, I. J. and Hart, I. R., Biological diversity in metastatic neoplasms: origins and implications, *Science,* 217, 988, 1982.
43. Talmadge, J. E., Wolman, S. R., and Fidler, I. J., Evidence for the clonal origin of spontaneous metastases, *Science,* 217, 361, 1982.
44. Poste, G., Doll, J., and Fidler, I. J., Interactions between clonal subpopulations affect the stability of the metastatic phenotype in polyclonal populations of the B16 melanoma cells, *Proc. Natl. Acad. Sci. U.S.A.,* 78, 6226, 1981.
45. Cifone, M. A. and Fidler, I. J., Increasing metastatic potential is associated with increasing genetic instability of clones isolated from murine neoplasms, *Proc. Natl. Acad. Sci. U.S.A.,* 78, 6949, 1981.
46. Hill, R. P., Chambers, A. F., Ling, V., and Harris, J. F., Dynamic heterogeneity: rapid generation of metastatic variants in mouse B16 melanoma cells, *Science,* 224, 998, 1984.
47. Barranco, S. C., Hanenelt, B. R., and Gea, E. L., Differential sensitivities of five rat hepatoma cell lines to anticancer drugs, *Cancer Res.,* 38, 656, 1978.
48. Hakansson, L. and Trope, C., Cell clones with different sensitivity to cytostatic drugs in methylcholanthrene-induced mouse sarcomas, *Acta Pathol. Microbiol. Scand. Sect. A,* 82, 41, 1974b.
49. Heppner, G. H., Dexter, D. L., DeNucci, T., Miller, F. R., and Calabresi, P., Heterogeneity in drug sensitivity among tumor cell subpopulations of a single mammary tumor, *Cancer Res.,* 38, 3758, 1978.
50. Lotan, R., Different susceptibilities of human melanoma and breast carcinoma cell lines to retinoic acid-induced growth inhibition, *Cancer Res.,* 39, 1014, 1979.
51. Trope, C., Aspergen, K., Kullander, S., and Astredt, B., Heterogeneous response of disseminated human ovarian cancers to cytostasis in vitro, *Acta Obstet. Gynecol. Scand.,* 58, 543, 1979.
52. Baylin, S. B., Clonal selection and heterogeneity of human solid neoplasms, in *Design of Models for Testing Cancer Therapeutic Agents,* Fidler, I. J. and White, R. J., Eds., Van Nostrand, New York, 1981, 50.
53. Tsuruo, T. and Fidler, I. J., Differences in drug sensitivity among tumor cells from parental tumors, selected variants, and spontaneous metastases, *Cancer Res.,* 41, 3058, 1981.
54. Abelof, M. D., Ettinger, D. S., Khouri, N. F., and Lenhard, R. E., Intensive induction therapy for small cell carcinoma of the lung, *Cancer Treat. Rep.,* 63, 519, 1979.
55. Livinston, R. B., Treatment of small cell carcinoma: evaluation and future directions, *Semin. Oncol.,* 5, 299, 1979.
56. Olsson, L. and Ebbensen, P., Natural polyclonality of spontaneous AKR leukemia and its consequence for so-called specific immunotherapy, *J. Natl. Cancer Inst.,* 62, 623, 1979.
57. Keller, R. and Jones, V. E., Role of activated macrophages and antibody in inhibition and enhancement of tumor growth in rats, *Lancet,* 2, 847, 1971.
58. Hibbs, J. B., Lambert, L. H., and Remington, J. S., Macrophage-mediated nonspecific cytotoxicity: possible role in tumor resistance, *Nature (London) New Biol.,* 235, 48, 1972a.
59. Cleveland, R. P., Meltzer, M. S., and Zbar, B., Tumor cytotoxicity in vitro by macrophages from mice infected with *Mycobacterium bovis* strain BCG, *J. Natl. Cancer Inst.,* 52, 1887, 1974.
60. Alexander, P. and Evans, R., Endotoxin and double stranded RNA render macrophages cytotoxic, *Nature (London),* 232, 76, 1971.
61. Hibbs, J. B., Jr., Taintor, R. R., Chapman, H. A., Jr., and Weinberg, J. B., Macrophage tumor killing: influence of the local environment, *Science,* 197, 279, 1977.
62. Doc, W. F. and Henson, P. M., Macrophage stimulation by bacterial lipopolysaccharides, *J. Exp. Med.,* 148, 544, 1978.
63. Pace, J. L. and Russell, S. W., Activation of mouse macrophages for tumor cell killing. I. Quantitative analysis of interactions between lymphokine and lipopolysaccharide, *J. Immunol.,* 126, 1863, 1981.
64. Peu, G., Polentarutti, N., Sessa, C., Mangioni, C., and Mantovani, A., Tumoricidal activity of macrophages isolated from human ascitic and solid ovarian carcinomas: augmentation by interferon, lymphokines and endotoxin, *Int. J. Cancer,* 28, 143, 1981.
65. Juv, D. and Chedid, L., Comparison between macrophage activation and enhancement of nonspecific resistance to tumors by mycobacterial immunoadjuvants, *Proc. Natl. Acad. Sci. U.S.A.,* 72, 4105, 1975.

66. Taniyama, T. and Holden, H. T., Direct augmentation of cytolytic activity of tumor-derived macrophages and macrophage cell lines by muramyl dipeptide, *Cell. Immunol.*, 48, 369, 1979.
67. Sone, S. and Fidler, I. J., In vitro activation of tumoricidal properties in rat alveolar macrophages by synthetic muramyl dipeptide encapsulated in liposomes, *Cell. Immunol.*, 57, 42, 1981a.
68. Kripke, M. L., Budmen, M. B., and Fidler, I. J., Production of specific macrophage-activating factor by lymphocytes from tumor-bearing mice, *Cell. Immunol.*, 30, 341, 1976.
69. Boraschi, D. and Tagliabui, A., Interferon-induced enhancement of macrophage-mediated tumor cytolysis and its difference from activation by lymphokines, *Eur. J. Immunol.*, 11, 110, 1981.
70. David, J. R., Macrophage activation by lymphocyte mediators, *Fed. Proc.*, 34, 1730, 1975.
71. Churchill, W. H., Piessens, W. F., Sulis, C. A., and David, J. R., Macrophages activated as suspension cultures with lymphocyte mediators devoid of antigens become cytotoxic for tumor cells, *J. Immunol.*, 115, 781, 1975.
72. Fidler, I. J. and Raz, A., The induction of tumoricidal capacities in mouse and rat macrophages by lymphokines, in *Lymphokines,* Pick, E., Ed., Academic Press, New York, 1981, 345.
73. Schultz, R. M., Papamatheakis, J. D., and Chirigos, M. A., Interferon: an inducer of macrophage activation by polyanions, *Science,* 197, 674, 1977.
74. Evans, R., Specific and nonspecific activation of macrophages. Activation of macrophages: proceedings of the Second Workshop Conference, Hoechst, Schlosf Reisensburg, 25-26 October, 1972, *Excerpta Med.*, 305, 1974.
75. Barna, B. P., Deodhar, S. D., Gautam, S., Yen-Lieberman, B., and Roberts, D., Macrophage activation and generation of tumoricidal activity by liposome-associated human C-reactive protein, *Cancer Res.*, 44, 305, 1984.
76. Munder, P. G., Weltzien, H. V., and Modelell, M., Lysolecithin analogs: a new class of immunopotentiators, in *Immunopathology,* Miescher, P. A., Ed., Grune & Stratton, New York, 1977, 411.
77. Tarnowski, G. S., Mountain, I. M., Stock, C. C., Munder, P. G., Weltzier, H. L., and Westphal, O., Effects of lysolecithin and analogs on mouse ascites tumors, *Cancer Res.*, 38, 339, 1978.
78. Hibbs, J. B., Jr., Discrimination between neoplastic and nonneoplastic cells in vitro by activated macrophages, *J. Natl. Cancer Inst.*, 53, 1487, 1974a.
79. Piessens, W. F. and Churchill, W. H., Jr., Macrophages activated in vitro with lymphocyte mediators kill neoplastic but not normal cells, *J. Immunol.*, 114, 1975.
80. Fidler, I. J., Recognition and destruction of target cells by tumoricidal macrophages, *Isr. J. Med.*, 14, 177, 1978b.
81. Fidler, I. J. and Kleinerman, E. S., Lymphokine-activated human blood monocytes destroy tumor cells but not normal cells under cocultivation conditions, *J. Clin. Oncol.*, 2, 937, 1984.
82. Kripke, M. L., Gruys, E., and Fidler, I. J., Metastatic heterogeneity of cells from an ultraviolet light-induced murine fibrosarcoma of recent origin, *Cancer Res.*, 38, 2962, 1978.
83. Fidler, I. J. and Cifone, M. A., Properties of metastatic and nonmetastatic cloned subpopulations of an ultraviolet-light-induced murine fibrosarcoma of recent origin, *Am. J. Pathol.*, 97, 633, 1979.
84. Reading, C. L., Kraemer, P. M., Miner, K. M., and Nicolson, G. L., In vivo and in vitro properties of malignant variants of RAW 117 metastatic murine lymphoma lymphosarcoma, *Clin. Exp. Met.*, 1, 135, 1983.
85. Miner, K. M., Klostergaard, J., Granger, G. A., and Nicolson, G. L., Differences in cytotoxic effects of activated murine peritoneal macrophages and J774 monocytic cells on metastatic variants of B16 melanoma, *J. Natl. Cancer Inst.*, 70, 717, 1983.
86. Fidler, I. J., Roblin, R. O., and Poste, G., In vitro tumoricidal activity of macrophages against virus-transformed lines with temperature-dependent transformed phenotypic characteristics, *Cell. Immunol.*, 38, 131, 1978b.
87. Giavazzi, R., Bucana, C. D., and Hart, I. R., Correlation of tumor growth inhibitory activity of macrophages exposed to Adriamycin and the Adriamycin sensitivity of the target tumor cells, *J. Natl. Cancer Inst.*, 73, 447, 1984.
88. Fogler, W. E. and Fidler, I. J., Nonselective destruction of murine neoplastic cells by syngeneic tumoricidal macrophages, *Cancer Res.*, 45, 14, 1985.
89. Fidler, I. J., Gersten, D. M., and Budmen, M. B., Characterization in vivo and in vitro of tumor cells selected for resistance to syngeneic lymphocyte-mediated cytotoxicity, *Cancer Res.*, 36, 3160, 1976.
90. Granger, G. A. and Weiser, R. S., Homograft target cells: specific destruction in vitro by contact interaction with immune macrophages, *Science,* 145, 1427, 1964.
91. Evans, R. and Alexander, P., Mechanism of immunologically specific killing of tumor cells by macrophages, *Nature (London),* 236, 168, 1972.
92. Keller, R., Cytostatic elimination of syngeneic rat tumor cells in vitro by nonspecifically activated macrophages, *J. Exp. Med.*, 138, 625, 1973.
93. Keller, R., Susceptibility of normal and transformed cell lines to cytostatic and cytocidal effects exerted by macrophages, *J. Natl. Cancer Inst.*, 56, 369, 1976.

94. Hibbs, J. B., Lambert, L. H., and Remington, J. S., Control of carcinogenesis: a possible role for the activated macrophage, *Science,* 177, 998, 1972b.

95. Hibbs, J. B., Jr., Macrophage nonimmunologic recognition: target cell factors related to contact inhibition, *Science,* 180, 868, 1973.

96. Meltzer, M. S., Tucker, R. W., Sanford, K. K., and Leonard, E. J., Interaction of BCG-activated macrophages with neoplastic and nonneoplastic cell lines in vitro: quantitation of the cytotoxic reaction by release of tritiated thymidine from prelabeled target cells, *J. Natl. Cancer Inst.,* 54, 1177, 1975b.

97. Norbury, K. and Fidler, I. J., In vitro tumor cell cytotoxicity by syngeneic mouse macrophages: methods for assaying cytotoxicity, *J. Immunol. Methods,* 7, 109, 1975.

98. Raz, A., Fogler, W. E., and Fidler, I. J., The effects of experimental conditions on the expression of in vitro mediated tumor cytotoxicity, *Cancer Immunol. Immunother.,* 7, 157, 1979.

99. Meltzer, M. S., Tucker, R. W., and Brever, A. C., Interaction of BCG-activated macrophages with neoplastic and nonneoplastic cell lines in vitro: cinemicrographic analysis, *Cell. Immunol.,* 17, 30, 1975a.

100. Bucana, C., Hoyer, L. C., Hobbs, B., Breesman, S., McDaniel, M., and Hanna, M. G., Jr., Morphological evidence for the translocation of lysosomal organelles from cytotoxic macrophages into the cytoplasm of tumor target cells, *Cancer Res.,* 36, 4444, 1976.

101. Hibbs, J. B., Jr., Heterocytolysis by macrophages activated by bacillus Calmette-Guerin: lysosome exocytosis into tumor cells, *Science,* 184, 468, 1974b.

102. Miller, M. L., Stimmett, J. D., and Clark, L. C., Jr., Ultrastructure of tumoricidal peritoneal exudate cells stimulated in vivo by perfluorochemical emulsions, *J. Reticuloendothel. Soc.,* 27, 105, 1980.

103. Kaplan, A. M., Brown, J., Collins, J. M., Morahan, P. S., and Snodgrass, M. J., Mechanisms of macrophage-mediated tumor cell cytotoxicity, *J. Immunol.,* 121, 1781, 1978.

104. Allison, A. C., Macrophage activation and nonspecific immunity, *Int. Rev. Exp. Pathol.,* 18, 303, 1978.

105. Aksamit, R. R. and Kim, K. J., Macrophage cell lines produce a cytotoxin, *J. Immunol.,* 122, 1785, 1979.

106. Currie, G. A. and Basham, C., Differential arginine dependence and the selective cytotoxic effects of activated macrophages for malignant cells in vitro, *Br. J. Cancer,* 39, 653, 1978.

107. McIvoc, K. L. and Weiser, R. S., Mechanisms of target cell destruction by alloimmune peritoneal macrophages. II. Release of a specific cytotoxin from interacting cells, *Immunology,* 20, 315, 1971.

108. Pipen, C. E. and McIvoc, K. L., Alloimmune peritoneal macrophages as specific effector cells: characterization of specific macrophage cytotoxin, *Cell. Immunol.,* 17, 423, 1975.

109. Sharma, S. F., Piessens, W. F., and Middlebrook, G., In vitro killing of tumor cells by soluble products of activated guinea pig peritoneal macrophages, *Cell. Immunol.,* 49, 379, 1980.

110. Drysdale, B., Zacharchuk, C. M., and Shin, H. S., Mechanism of macrophage-mediated cytotoxicity: production of a soluble cytotoxic factor, *J. Immunol.,* 131, 2362, 1983.

111. Ferluga, J., Schorlemmer, H. U., Baptista, C. C., and Allison, A. C., Production of the complement cleavage product, C3a, by activated macrophages and its tumorilytic effects, *Clin. Exp. Immunol.,* 31, 512, 1978.

112. Stadecker, M. J., Calderon, J., Karnovsky, M. J., and Unanue, E. R., Synthesis and release of thymidine by macrophage, *J. Immunol.,* 119, 1738, 1978.

113. Nathan, C. F., Brukner, L. H., Silverstein, S. C., and Cohn, Z. A., Extracellular cytolysis by activated macrophages and granulocytes. I. Pharmacologic triggering of effector cells and the release of hydrogen peroxide, *J. Exp. Med.,* 149, 84, 1979A.

114. Nathan, C. F., Silverstein, S. C., Brukner, L. H., and Cohn, Z. A., Extracellular cytolysis by activated macrophages and granulocytes. II. Hydrogen peroxide as a mediator of cytotoxicity, *J. Exp. Med.,* 149, 100, 1979B.

115. Adams, D. O., Effector mechanism of cytolytically activated macrophages. I. Secretion of neutral proteases and effect of protease inhibitors, *J. Immunol.,* 124, 286, 1980.

116. Adams, D. O., Kao, K. J., Farb, R., and Pizzol, S. V., Effector mechanisms of cytolytically activated macrophages. II. Secretion of a cytolytic factor by activated macrophages and its relationship to secreted neutral proteases, *J. Immunol.,* 124, 293, 1980.

117. Cohn, Z. A., The activation of mononuclear phagocytes: fact, fancy and future, *J. Immunol.,* 121, 813, 1978.

118. North, R. J., The concept of the activated macrophages, *J. Immunol.,* 121, 806, 1978.

119. Poste, G., Kirsh, R., and Fidler, I. J., Cell surface receptors for lymphokines. I. The possible role of glycolipids as receptors for macrophage migration inhibitor factor (MIF) and macrophage activating factor (MAF), *Cell. Immunol.,* 44, 71, 1979.

120. Poste, G., Kirsh, R., Fogler, W. E., and Fidler, I. J., Activation of tumoricidal properties in mouse macrophages by lymphokines encapsulated in liposomes, *Cancer Res.,* 39, 881, 1979B.

121. Piessens, W. F., Remold, H. G., and David, J. R., Increased responsiveness to macrophage-activating factor (MAF) after alteration of macrophage membranes, *J. Immunol.*, 118, 2078, 1977.

122. Celada, A., Gray, P. W., Rinderknecht, E., and Schreiber, R., Evidence for a gamma-interferon receptor that regulates macrophage tumoricidal activity, *J. Exp. Med.*, 160, 55, 1984.

123. Sone, S., Poste, G., and Fidler, I. J., Rat alveolar macrophages are susceptible to free and liposome-encapsulated lymphokines, *J. Immunol.*, 124, 2197, 1980.

124. Fidler, I. J., Raz, A., Fogler, W. E., Hoyer, L. C., and Poste, G., The role of plasma membrane receptors and the kinetics of macrophage activation by lymphokines encapsulated in liposomes, *Cancer Res.*, 41, 495, 1981B.

125. Fogler, W. E., Talmadge, J., and Fidler, I. J., The activation of tumoricidal properties in macrophages of endotoxin responder and nonresponder mice by liposome-encapsulated immunomodulators, *J. Reticuloendothel. Soc.*, 33, 165, 1983.

126. Kleinerman, E. S., Schroit, A. J., Fogler, W. E., and Fidler, I. J., Tumoricidal activity of human monocytes activated in vitro by free and liposome-encapsulated human lymphokines, *J. Clin. Invest.*, 72, 304, 1983.

127. Ellouz, F., Adam, A., Ciorbaru, R., and Lederer, E., Minimal structural requirements for adjuvant activity of bacterial peptidoglycan derivatives, *Biochem. Biophys. Res. Commun.*, 59, 1317, 1974.

128. Kotani, S., Watanabe, Y., Shimono, T., Narita, T., Kato, K., Stewart-Tull, D. E. S., Kinoshita, F., Yokogawa, K., Kawata, S., Shiba, T., Kusumoto, S., and Tarumi, Y., Immunoadjuvant activities of cell walls, their water-soluble fractions and peptidoglycan subunits, prepared from various gram-positive bacteria, and of synthetic N-acetyl-muramyl peptides, *Z. Immun. Forsch. Exp. Ther.*, 149, 302, 1975.

129. Tenu, J. P., Roche, A. C., Yapo, A., Kieda, C., Monsigny, M., and Petit, J. F., Absence of cell surface receptors for muramyl peptides in mouse peritoneal macrophages, *Biol. Cell*, 144, 157, 1982.

130. Fogler, W. E. and Fidler, I. J., The activation of tumoricidal properties in human blood monocytes by muramyl peptides requires a specific requires a specific intracellular interaction, *J. Immunol.*, 136, 2311, 1986.

131. Chapes, S. K. and Haskill, S., Role of *Corynebacterium parvum* in the activation of peritoneal macrophages. I. Association between intracellular *C. parvum* and cytotoxic macrophages, *Cell. Immunol.*, 70, 65., 1982.

132. Fidler, I. J., Sone, S., Fogler, W. E., and Barnes, Z., Eradication of spontaneous metastases and activation of alveolar macrophages by intravenous injection of liposomes containing muramyl dipeptide, *Proc. Natl. Acad. Sci. U.S.A.*, 78, 1680, 1981.

133. Schroit, A. J. and Fidler, I. J., Effects of liposome structure and lipid composition on the activation of tumoricidal properties of macrophages by liposomes containing muramyl dipeptide, *Cancer Res.*, 42, 161, 1982.

134. Fidler, I. J., Sone, S., Fogler, W. E., Smith, D., Braun, D. G., Tarcsay, L., Gisler, R. H., and Schroit, A. J., Efficacy of liposomes containing a lipophilic muramyl dipeptide derivative for activating the tumoricidal properties of alveolar macrophages in vivo, *J. Biol. Resp. Modif.*, 1, 43, 1982.

135. Phillips, N. C., Moras, M. L., Chedid, L., Lefrancier, P., and Bernard, J. M., Activation of alveolar macrophage tumoricidal activity and eradication of experimental metastases by freeze-dried liposomes containing a lipophilic muramyl dipeptide derivative, *Cancer Res.*, 45, 128, 1985.

136. Lopez-Berestein, G., Mehta, K., Mehta, R., Juliano, R. L., and Hersh, E. M., The activation of human monocytes by liposome-encapsulated muramyl dipeptide analogues, *J. Immunol.*, 130, 1500, 1983.

137. Sone, S., Musuura, S., Ogawara, M., and Tsubura, E., Potentiating effect of muramyl dipeptide and its lipophilic analog encapsulated in liposomes on tumor cell killing by human monocytes, *J. Immunol.*, 1984.

138. Kleinerman, E. S., Erickson, K. L., Schroit, A. J., Fogler, W. E., and Fidler, I. J., Activation of tumoricidal properties in human blood monocytes by liposomes containing lipophilic muramyl tripeptide, *Cancer Res.*, 43, 2010, 1983.

139. Koff, W. C., Fidler, I. J., Showalter, S. D., Chakrabarty, M. K., Hampar, B., Ceccorulli, L. M., and Kleinerman, E. S., Human blood monocytes activated by immunomodulators in liposomes lyse herpes virus-infected but not normal cells, *Science*, 224, 1007, 1984.

140. Kleinschmidt, W. J. and Schultz, R. M., Similarities of murine gamma interferon and the lymphokine that renders macrophages cytotoxic, *J. Interferon Res.*, 2, 291, 1982.

141. Schultz, R. M., Synergistic activation of macrophages by lymphokine and lipopolysaccharide: evidence for lymphokine as the primer and interferon as the trigger, *J. Interferon Res.*, 2, 459, 1982.

142. Kleinerman, E. S., Zicht, R., Sarin, P. S., Gallo, R. C., and Fidler, I. J., Constitutive production and release of a lymphokine with macrophage-activating factor activity distinct from gamma-interferon by a human T-cell leukemia virus-positive cell line, *Cancer Res.*, 44, 4470, 1984.

143. Ruco, L. P. and Meltzer, M. S., Macrophage activation for tumor cytotoxicity: development of macrophage cytotoxic activity requires completion of a sequence of short-lived intermediary reactions, *J. Immunol.*, 121, 2035, 1978.

144. Sone, S. and Fidler, I. J., Synergistic activation by lymphokines and muramyl dipeptide of tumoricidal properties in rat alveolar macrophages, *J. Immunol.*, 125, 2454, 1980.

145. Fidler, I. J. and Schroit, A. J., Synergism between lymphokines and muramyl dipeptide encapsulated in liposomes: in situ activation of macrophages and therapy of spontaneous cancer metastases, *J. Immunol.*, 133, 515, 1984.

146. Ruco, L. P. and Meltzer, M. S., Macrophage activation for tumor cytotoxicity: tumoricidal activity by macrophages from C3H/JeJ mice requires at least two activation stimuli, *Cell. Immunol.*, 41, 35, 1978.

147. Saiki, I. and Fidler, I. J., Synergistic activation by recombinant mouse gamma-interferon and muramyl dipeptide of tumoricidal properties in mouse macrophages, *J. Immunol.*, 135, 684, 1985.

148. Saiki, I., Sone, S., Fogler, W. E., Kleinerman, E. S., Lopez-Berestein, G., and Fidler, I. J., Synergism between human recombinant gamma-interferon and muramyl dipeptide encapsulated in liposomes for activation of antitumor properties in human blood monocytes, *Cancer Res.*, 45, 6188, 1985.

149. Fidler, I. J., Fogler, W. E., Kleinerman, E. S., and Saiki, I., Abrogation of species specificity for activation of tumoricidal properties in macrophages by recombinant mouse or human gamma interferon encapsulated in liposomes, *J. Immunol.*, 135, 4289, 1985.

150. Taffet, S. M., Pace, J. L., and Russell, S. W., Lymphokine maintains macrophage activation for tumor cell killing by interfering with the negative regulatory effect of prostaglandin E_2, *J. Immunol.*, 127, 121, 1981.

151. Taffet, S. M. and Russell, S. W., Macrophage-mediated tumor cell killing: regulation of expression of cytolytic activity by prostaglandin E, *J. Immunol.*, 126, 424, 1981.

152. Drysdale, B. E. and Shin, H. S., Activation of macrophages for tumor cell cytotoxicity: identification of indomethacin sensitive and insensitive pathways, *J. Immunol.*, 127, 760, 1981.

153. Koff, W. C. and Dunegan, M. A., Modulation of macrophage-mediated tumoricidal activity by neuropeptides and neurohormones, *J. Immunol.*, 135, 350, 1985.

154. Fidler, I. J., The MAF dilemma, *Lymphokine Res.*, 3, 51, 1984.

155. Kay, M. M. B., Mechanism of removal of senescent cells by human macrophages in situ, *Proc. Natl. Acad. Sci. U.S.A.*, 72, 3521, 1975.

156. Macdonald, R. A., MacSween, R. N. M., and Pechet, G. S., Iron metabolism by reticuloendothelial cells in vitro: physical and chemical conditions, lipotrope deficiency, and acute inflammation, *Lab. Invest.*, 21, 236, 1969.

157. Day, A. J., The macrophage system, lipid metabolism and atherosclerosis, *J. Atheroscler. Res.*, 4, 117, 1964.

158. Cohn, Z. A., The structure and function of monocytes and macrophages, *Adv. Immunol.*, 9, 163, 1968.

159. Van Furth, R., *Mononuclear phagocytes in immunity, infection and pathology*, Blackwell Scientific, Oxford, 1975.

160. Nathan, C. F., Murray, H. W., and Cohn, A. Z., Current concepts: the macrophage as an effetor cell, *N. Engl. J. Med.*, 303, 622, 1980.

161. Nelson, D. S., *Immunobiology of the Macrophage,* Academic Press, New York, 1976.

162. Fink, M. A., *The Macrophage in Neoplasia,* Academic Press, New York, 1976.

163. James, K., McBride, B., and Stuart, A., *The Macrophage and Cancer,* University of Edinburg Press, Edinburg, 1977.

164. Evans, R. and Alexander, P., Mechanisms of extracellular killing of nucleated mammalian cells by macrophages, in *The Immunobiology of the Macrophage,* Nelson, D. S., Ed., Academic Press, New York, 1976, p. 562.

165. Lurie, H., *Resistance of Tuberculosis: Experimental Studies in Native and Acquired Defense Mechanisms,* Harvard University Press, Cambridge, 1964.

166. Droller, M. J. and Remmington, J. S., A role for the macrophage in in vivo and in vitro resistance to murine bladder tumor cell growth, *Cancer Res.*, 35, 49, 1975.

167. Norbury, K. and Kripke, M. L., Ultraviolet-induced carcinogenesis in mice treated with silica, trypan blue or pyran copolymer, *J. Reticuloendothel. Soc.*, 26, 827, 1979.

168. Jones, P. D. E. and Castro, J. E., Immunological mechanisms in metastatic spread and the antimetastatic effects of *C. parvum, Br. J. Cancer,* 35, 519, 1977.

169. Sadler, T. E., Jones, D. D. E., and Castro, J. E., The effects of altered phagocytic activity on growth of primary and metastatic tumors, in *The Macrophage and Cancer,* McBride, J. F. and Stuart, A., Eds., Econoprint, Edinburg, 115, 1979.

170. Mantovani, A., Giavazzi, R., Polentanitti, N., Spreafico, F., and Gavattinni, S., Divergent effects of macrophage toxins on growth of primary tumors and lung metastases in mice, *Int. J. Cancer,* 25, 617, 1980.

171. Fidler, I. J., Inhibition of pulmonary metastasis by intravenous injection of specifically activated macrophages, *Cancer Res.*, 34, 1074, 1974B.
172. Liotta, L. A., Gattozzi, C., Kleinerman, J., and Saidel, G., Reduction of tumor cell entry into vessels by BCG-activated macrophages, *Br. J. Cancer*, 36, 639, 1977.
173. Fidler, I. J., Fogler, W. E., and Connor, J., The rationale for the treatment of established experimental micrometastases with the injection of tumoricidal macrophages, in *Immunobiology and Immunotherapy of Cancer*, Terry, W. D. and Yamamura, Y., Eds., Elsevier, Amsterdam, 361, 1979A.
174. Den Otter, W., Dullens, H. F. J., Van Lovern, H., and Pels, E., Antitumor effectors of macrophages injected into animals: a review, in *The Macrophage and Cancer*, James, K., McBride, B., and Stuart, A., Eds., Econoprint, Edinburg, 119, 1977.
175. Blamey, R. W., Crosby, D. L., and Baker, J. M., Reticuloendothelial activity during the growth of rat sarcomas, *Cancer Res.*, 29, 335, 1969.
176. Old, L. J., Clarke, D. A., Benacerraf, B., and Goldsmith, M., The reticuloendothelial system and the neoplastic process, *Science*, 88, 164, 1960.
177. Rhodes, J., Altered expression of human monocyte Fc receptors in malignant disease, *Nature (London)*, 265, 253, 1977.
178. Rhodes, J., Resistance of tumor cells to macrophages, *Cancer Immunol. Immunother.*, 7, 211, 1980.
179. Bernstein, I. D., Zbar, B., and Rapp, H. J., Impaired inflammatory response in tumor-bearing guinea pigs, *J. Natl. Cancer Inst.*, 49, 1641, 1972.
180. Eccles, S. A. and Alexander, P., Sequestration of macrophages in growing tumors and its effect on the immunological capacity of the host, *Br. J. Cancer*, 30, 42, 1974A.
181. Meltzer, M. S. and Stevenson, M. M., Macrophage function in tumor-bearing mice: tumoricidal and chemotactic response of macrophages activated by infection with *Mycobacterium bovis*, strain BCG, *J. Immunol.*, 118, 2176, 1977.
182. Meltzer, M. S. and Stevenson, M. M., Macrophage function in tumor-bearing mice: dissociation of phagocytic and chemotactic responsiveness, *Cell. Immunol.*, 35, 99, 1978.
183. Normann, S. J. and Sorkin, E., Cell-specific defect in monocyte function during tumor growth, *J. Natl. Cancer Inst.*, 57, 135, 1976.
184. Snyderman, R., Pike, M. C., Blaylock, B. L., and Weinstein, P., Effect of neoplasms on inflammation: depression of macrophage accumulation after tumor implantation, *J. Immunol.*, 116, 585, 1976.
185. Sone, S. and Fidler, I. J., Activation of rat alveolar macrophages to the tumoricidal state in the presence of progressively growing pulmonary metastases, *Cancer Res.*, 41, 2401, 1981B.
186. Mantovani, A., Effects on in vitro tumor growth of murine macrophages isolated from sarcoma lines differing in immunogenicity and metastasizing capacity, *Int. J. Cancer*, 22, 741, 1978.
187. Russell, S. W. and McIntosh, A. T., Macrophages isolated from regressing Moloney sarcomas are more cytotoxic than those recovered from progressing sarcomas, *Nature (London)*, 268, 69, 1977.
188. Loveless, S. E. and Heppner, G. H., Tumor associated macrophages of mouse mammary tumors. I. Differential cytotoxicity of macrophages from metastatic and nonmetastatic tumors, *J. Immunol.*, 131, 2074, 1983.
189. Evans, R., Tumor macrophages in host immunity to malignancies, in *The Macrophage in Neoplasia*, Fink, M. A., Ed., Academic Press, New York, 1976, 27.
190. Eccles, S. A. and Alexander, P., Macrophage content of tumors in relationship to metastatic spread, *Nature (London)*, 250, 667, 1974B.
191. Eccles, S. A., Macrophages and cancer, in *Immunological Aspects of Cancer*, Castro, J. E., Ed., MTP Press, Lancaster, England, 1978, 123.
192. Talmadge, J. E., Key, M., and Fidler, I. J., Macrophage content of metastatic and nonmetastatic rodent neoplasms, *J. Immunol.*, 126, 2245, 1981.
193. Nash, J. R. G., Price, J. E., and Tarin, D., Macrophage content and colony-forming potential in mouse mammary carcinomas, *Br. J. Cancer*, 45, 478, 1981.
194. Mahoney, K. H., Fulton, A. M., and Heppner, G. H., Tumor-associated macrophages of mouse mammary tumors. II. Differential distribution of macrophages from metastatic and nonmetastatic tumors, *J. Immunol.*, 131, 2079, 1983.
195. Evans, R. and Eidler, D. M., Macrophage accumulation in transplanted tumors is not dependent on host immune responsiveness or presence of tumor-associated rejection antigens, *J. Reticuloendothel. Soc.*, 30, 425, 1981.
196. Evans, R. and Lawler, E. M., Macrophage content and immunogenicity of C56BL/6J and BALB/cByJ methylcholanthrene-induced sarcomas, *Int. J. Cancer*, 26, 831, 1980.
197. Dvorak, H. R., Dickersin, G. R., Dvorak, A. M., Manseau, E. J., and Pyne, K., Human breast carcinoma: fibrin deposits and desmoplasia. Inflammatory cell type and distribution in microvasculature and infarction, *J. Natl. Cancer Inst.*, 67, 335, 1981.
198. Key, M., Talmadge, J. E., and Fidler, I. J., Lack of correlation between the progressive growth of spontaneous metastases and their content of infiltrating macrophages, *J. Reticuloendothel. Soc.*, 32, 387, 1982.

199. Mantovani, A., In vitro effects on tumor cells of macrophages isolated from an early-passage chemically-induced murine sarcoma and from its spontaneous metastases, *Int. J. Cancer,* 27, 221, 1981.
200. Allison, A. C., Model of action of immunological adjuvants, *J. Reticuloendothel. Soc.,* 26, 619, 1979.
201. Chedid, L., Audibert, F., and Johnson, A. G., Biological activities of muramyl dipeptide, a synthetic glycopeptide analogous to bacterial immunoregulating agents, *Prog. Allergy,* 25, 63, 1978.
202. Fogler, W. E. and Fidler, I. J., Modulation of the immune response by muramyl dipeptide, in *Immune Modulation Agents and Their Mechanisms,* Chirigos, M. A. and Fenichel, R. L., Eds., Marcel Dekker, New York, 1984, 499.
203. Parant, M., Parant, F., Chedid, L., Yalo, A., Petit, J. F., and Lederer, E., Fate of the synthetic immunoadjuvant, muramyl dipeptide, (^{14}C-labeled) in the mouse, *Int. J. Immunopharmacol.,* 1, 35, 1978.
204. Ambler, L. and Hudson, A. M., Pharmacokinetics and metabolism of muramyl dipeptide and normuramyl dipeptide (^{3}H-labeled) in the mouse, *Int. J. Immunopharmacol.,* 6, 133, 1984.
205. Yoshida, T. and Cohen, S., Lymphokine activity in vivo in relation to circulating monocyte levels and delayed skin reactivity, *J. Immunol.,* 122, 1540, 1972.
206. Papermaster, B. W., Holterman, O. A., Rosner, D., Klein, E., Dao, T., and Djerassi, I., Regressions produced in breast cancer lesions by a lymphokine fraction from a human lymphoid cell line, *Res. Commun. Chem. Pathol. Pharmacol.,* 8, 413, 1974.
207. Salvin, S. B., Youngner, Y. S., Nishio, J., and Neta, R., Tumor suppression by a lymphokine release into the circulation of mice with delayed hypersensitivity, *J. Natl. Cancer Inst.,* 55, 1233, 1975.
208. Donohue, J. H. and Rosenburg, S. A., The fate of interleukin-2 after in vivo administration, *J. Immunol.,* 130, 2203, 1983.
209. Poste, G. and Kirsh, R., Rapid decay of tumoricidal activity and loss of responsiveness to lymphokines in inflammatory macrophage, *Cancer Res.,* 39, 2582, 1979.
210. Schroit, A. J., Hart, I. R., Madsen, J., and Fidler, I. J., Selective delivery of drugs encapsulated in liposomes: natural targeting to macrophages involved in various disease states, *J. Biol. Resp. Modif.,* 2, 97, 1983.
211. Poste, G., Kirsh, R., and Bugelski, P., Liposomes as a drug delivery system in cancer therapy, in *New Approaches to Cancer Chemotherapy,* Academic Press, New York, 1984, 165.
212. Allison, A. C. and Gregoriadis, G., Liposomes as immunological adjuvants, *Nature (London),* 252, 252, 1979
213. Fidler, I. J., Raz, A., Fogler, W. E., Kirsh, R., Bugelski, P., and Poste, G., Design of liposomes to improve delivery of macrophage-augmenting agents to alveolar macrophages, *Cancer Res.,* 40, 4460, 1980.
214. Hart, I. R., Fogler, W. E., Poste, G., and Fidler, I. J., Toxicity studies of liposome-encapsulated immunomodulators administered intravenously to dogs and mice, *Cancer Immunol. Immunother.,* 10, 157, 1981.
215. Fogler, W. E., Raz, A., and Fidler, I. J., In situ activation of murine macrophages by liposomes containing lymphokines, *Cell. Immunol.,* 53, 214.
216. Fidler, I. J., Therapy of spontaneous metastases by intravenous injection of liposomes containing lymphokines, *Science,* 208, 1469, 1980.
217. Griswold, D. P., Jr., Consideration of the subcutaneously implanted B16 melanoma as a screening model for potential anticancer agents, *Cancer Chemother.,* 3, 315, 1972.
218. Fogler, W. E., Wade, R., Brundish, and Fidler, I. J., Distribution and fate of free and liposome-encapsulated (^{3}H)nor-muramyl dipeptide and (^{3}H)muramyl tripeptide phosphatidylethanolamine in mice, *J. Immunol.,* in press.
219. Fogler, W. E. and Fidler, I. J., In situ activation of tumoricidal properties in murine alveolar macrophages following the systemic administration of muramyl dipeptide encapsulated within liposomes, *Fed. Proc.,* 40, 761, 1981.
220. Fidler, I. J., Barnes, Z., Fogler, W. E., Kirsh, R., Bugelski, P., and Poste, G., Involvement of macrophages in the eradication of established metastases produced by intravenous injection of liposomes containing macrophage activators, *Cancer Res.,* 42, 496, 1982A.
221. Fidler, I. J., The in situ induction of tumoricidal activity in alveolar macrophages by liposomes containing muramyl dipeptide is a thymus-independent process, *J. Immunol.,* 127, 1719, 1981.
222. Key, M. E., Talmadge, J. E., Fogler, W. E., Bucana, C., and Fidler, I. J., Isolation of tumoricidal macrophages from lung melanoma metastases of mice treated systemically with liposomes containing a lipophilic derivative of muramyl dipeptide, *J. Natl. Cancer Inst.,* 69, 1189, 1982.
223. Deodhar, S. D., Barna, B. P., Edinger, M., and Chiang, T., Inhibition of lung metastases by liposomal immunotherapy in a murine fibrosarcoma model, *J. Biol. Res. Modif.,* 1, 27, 1982.
224. Deodhar, S. D., James, K., Chiang, T., Edinger, M., and Barna, B., Inhibition of lung metastases in mice bearing a malignant fibrosarcoma by treatment with liposomes containing human c-reactive protein, *Cancer Res.,* 42, 5084, 1982.

225. Thombre, P. and Deodhar, S. D., Inhibition of liver metastases in murine colon adenocarcinoma by liposomes containing human c-reactive protein or crude lymphokine, *Cancer Immunol. Immunother.*, 16, 145, 1984.
226. Schroit, A. J. and Fidler, I. J., The design of liposomes for delivery of immunomodulators to host defense cells, in *Medical Applications of Liposomes,* Yagi, K., Ed., Japan Scientific Societies Press, Japan, in press.
227. Lopez-Berestein, G., Milas, L., Hunter, N., Mehta, K., Hersh, E. M., Kurahara, C. G., Vanderpas, M., and Eppstein, D. A., Prophylaxis and treatment of experimental lung metastases in mice after treatment with liposome-encapsulated 6-O-stearoyl-N-acetylmuramyl-L-α-aminobutyryl-D-isoglutamine, *Clin. Exp. Met.,* 2, 127, 1984.
228. Pabst, M. J., Cummings, N. P., Shiba, T., Kusumoto, S., and Kotani, S., Lipophilic derivative of muramyl dipeptide is more active than muramyl dipeptide in priming macrophages to release superoxide anion, *Infect. Immun.,* 29, 617, 1980.
229. Fidler, I. J., Sone, S., Fogler, W. E., Smith, D., Braun, D. G., Tarcsay, L., Gisler, R. H., and Schroit, A. J., Efficacy of liposomes containing a lipophilic muramyl dipeptide derivative for activating the tumoricidal properties of alveolar macrophages in vivo, *J. Biol. Resp. Modif.,* 1, 43, 1982B.
230. Raz, A., Bucana, C., Fogler, W. E., Poste, G., and Fidler, I. J., Biochemical, morphological, and ultrastructural studies on the uptake of liposomes by murine macrophages, *Cancer Res.,* 41, 487, 1981.
231. Fidler, I. J. and Poste, G., Macrophage-mediated destruction of malignant tumor cells and new strategies for the therapy of metastatic disease, *Springer Semin. Immunopathol.,* 5, 161, 1982.

Chapter 11

SUCCESSFUL ADOPTIVE IMMUNOTHERAPY OF ESTABLISHED METASTASES WITH LYMPHOKINE ACTIVATED KILLER CELLS AND RECOMBINANT INTERLEUKIN-2

J. J. Mulé and S. A. Rosenberg

TABLE OF CONTENTS

I. BACKGROUND

In a 1977 review of the adoptive immunotherapy of cancer, Rosenberg and Terry[1] summarized the evidence that the adoptive transfer of immunologically reactive lymphoid cells to the tumor-bearing host could mediate the regression of established tumors in animal models. It has generally been assumed that the most effective cells for adoptive immunotherapy of cancer would be those with exquisite specific reactivity to the tumor antigens present on cancer cells. Indeed, the i.v. infusion of fresh (or cultured), specifically sensitized T-lymphocytes has been shown to mediate the regression of established transplantable tumors in the mouse, rat, and guinea pig.[2-8] Virtually all prior attempts to perform adoptive immunotherapy of established experimental tumors have utilized highly immunogenic, well-defined tumors to which specifically immune cells can easily be raised.[1] These studies have established the principle that the infusion of a sufficient number of specifically immune lymphoid cells is capable of mediating the regression of established primary tumor, as well as tumor metastases, and have elucidated the factors involved in the successful application of this approach. Experimental models utilizing adoptive immunotherapy, however, have been carefully selected.[3,9-13] Specifically immune cells cannot be raised against all tumors and in the absence of specific immunization procedures for a given tumor this approach is not applicable. In general, animals have been hyperimmunized to the tumors by repeated challenges with tumor often in conjunction with immune adjuvants. These approaches are rarely feasible or effective in the human.

An analysis of successful adoptive immunotherapy reveals several factors that seem essential for successful treatment. Four of the most important factors are

1. Obtaining highly sensitized cells with specific antitumor reactivity.
2. Obtaining large numbers of sensitized cells (at least 10^8 cells to treat a 1 cm diameter tumor in a mouse).
3. Use of syngeneic cells for therapy.
4. The elimination of suppressor cells in the tumor-bearing host that will prevent the action of adoptively transferred cells.[14-16]

Early attempts at adoptive immunotherapy of human tumors, however, fall far short of meeting each of the above four criteria.

When one considers the very poor (or absence of) immunogenicity of human tumors, it is likely that the incidence of immune lymphocytes specifically reactive against these tumor antigens will be very low and that these cells will be difficult to identify and isolate. In addition, the use of human mixed lymphocyte-tumor cell cultures has not been effective in generating specifically sensitized lymphocytes with antitumor activity.[17] Thus, these factors have limited the applicability of this approach to the treatment of humans with cancer. We have published several reviews[18-20] pertaining to work from our laboratory examining lymphoid cells with specific reactivity to unique target antigens on virally or chemically induced tumors and the value of these cells in adoptive immunotherapy. Thus, we will not further elaborate on this topic in this chapter and will concentrate, rather, on our more recent work with nonspecifically activated lymphoid cells in the immunotherapy of established cancer metastases.

A. Lymphokine Activated Killer Cells

In 1980, we explored alternative approaches to generate nonspecifically activated cells with a high degree of antitumor reactivity. We first described that the incubation of murine and human lymphocytes in crude supernatants containing the lymphokine, IL-2 led to the generation of cells with the capacity to lyse fresh, noncultured autologous primary and metastatic cancer cells but not fresh normal cells, in short-term ^{51}Gr

Table 1

GENERATION OF MURINE LAK CELLS

| | C57BL/6 Splenocyte effector cells | | |
Target	Fresh (uncultured)	Cultured in mediam % lysis (± SEM)[a]	Cultured in IL-2
MCA-102 sarcoma	1 ± 1	2 ± 2	53 ± 2
MCA-106 sarcoma	3 ± 1	4 ± 1	53 ± 1
EL-4 lymphoma	−20 ± 2	−18 ± 1	43 ± 2
Normal splenocyte	−12 ± 3	−20 ± 5	8 ± 2
YAC	20 ± 1	8 ± 1	72 ± 1

[a]   100:1 effector:target.

From Rosenstein, M. et al., *Cancer Res.,* 44, 1946, 1984. With permission.

release assays.[21,22] In later studies using highly purified natural IL-2 and then recombinant derived IL-2 we showed that IL-2 was the lymphokine solely responsible for the generation of these lytic cells.[23,24] These activated lymphoid cells, which we have termed LAK cells, have been extensively characterized in both the human and mouse.[25-27] Much has been learned concerning LAK cells and the nature of this lytic system has been the subject of several overviews.[28-30]

Based upon criteria that include the cell surface phenotypes of precursor and effector cells, the spectrum and specificity of targets lysed and responsiveness to various biological response modifiers, LAK cells appear to represent a lytic system distinct from that of NK cells and cytotoxic T-lymphoid cells, although this is an area of some controversy. The relationship of LAK cells to other forms of anomalous cytotoxicity induced in vitro by a variety of other techniques, such as incubation with lectins,[31] pooled allogeneic stimulation,[32-34] or incubation in heterologous serum,[35] is unclear, although it is possible that IL-2 stimulation represents a final common pathway for generating these lytic activities in lymphocytes in vitro.

An example of the ability of IL-2 to generate LAK cells in the mouse is shown in Table 1.[25] In this experiment, splenocytes from C57BL/6 mice were tested against a variety of target cells for their ability to lyse tumor and normal syngeneic cells. The lytic activity of the splenocytes was tested before and after incubation in medium containing IL-2. Fresh uncultured splenocytes were capable of lysing the cultured YAC target, indicating that they had some NK cell activity. Fresh methylcholanthrene-induced sarcomas (MCA-102 and MCA-106) and the syngeneic EL-4 lymphoma were not lysed by these fresh splenocytes, indicating that they were resistant to lysis by NK cells. However, culture of these fresh splenocytes in IL-2 for 5 days generated LAK cells that were capable of killing the MCA-102 and MCA-106 sarcoma, the EL-4 lymphoma and YAC cells, but not normal lymphocytes. None of these targets were lysed by normal C57BL/6 splenocytes cultured in complete medium (without IL-2) for 5 days. The biologic role of these LAK cells is not known, but we have hypothesized that they may play a role in immune surveillance against transformed cells.[19] Because LAK cells are easily generated and show broad tumor specificity, these cells are logical candidates for use in adoptive immunotherapy.

The ability to use these cells in in vivo adoptive immunotherapy experiments, however, depended on the availability of large amounts of IL-2. In addition to the IL-2 needed to activate LAK cells, the exquisite dependence of these cells on the continued presence of IL-2 for their survival suggested that IL-2 administration to mice receiving

Table 2
LAK CELLS PLUS RECOMBINANT IL-2 MARKEDLY REDUCE THE NUMBER OF ARTIFICIALLY INDUCED, ESTABLISHED PULMONARY METASTASES OF B16 MELANOMA

Treatment group	No. of metastases per mouse	Mean	p^a
HBSS	250,250,151,129,114	179	—
RIL-2	250,250, 57, 26, 23	121	0.34
LAK cells + HBSS	250,250, 73, 42, 12	126	0.34
LAK cells + RIL-2	22, 22, 7, 7, 4	12	0.01

a Wilcoxon rank sum test of treated groups compared to group receiving HBSS alone (two-sided).

From Mulé, J. J. et al., *Cancer Res.*, 46, 676, 1985. With permission.

LAK cells would also be required. Moreover, since IL-2 was the sole activating agent responsible for the generation of LAK cells, it was further hypothesized that the systemic administration of this lymphokine may induce these cells directly in vivo. Donohue and Rosenberg[36] had shown that the serum half-life of IL-2 was only 2 min and thus large amounts of IL-2 were required to obtain sustained bioavailability for in vivo experiments.

The isolation of a human IL-2 DNA clone from the JURKAT cell line by Taniguchi et al. in 1983 provided the key to the production of large amounts of IL-2.[37] In 1984, Rosenberg et al. described the isolation of additional DNA clones coding for IL-2 from both the JURKAT cell line as well as from peripheral blood lymphocytes, the expression of these genes in the bacteria *Escherichia coli,* the purification to homogeneity of the IL-2 protein which appeared to be approximately 5% of all of the *E. coli* proteins, and a series of immunologic studies demonstrating the biologic equivalence of this recombinant human IL-2 with IL-2 obtained from natural sources.[24] This recombinant IL-2 was effective in the generation of LAK cells from murine and human lymphocytes in vitro and was well tolerated when injected intraperitoneally into mice.

Utilizing this recombinant IL-2 a variety of animal models were established to test the efficacy of LAK cells in the immunotherapy of established murine malignancies.[38-42] In each of these models tumor was established in either the lung or liver prior to instituting therapy.

II. SUCCESSFUL REDUCTION OF ESTABLISHED LUNG METASTASES WITH LYMPHOKINE-ACTIVATED KILLER CELLS PLUS RECOMBINANT IL-2

To study the effect of LAK cell therapy on established pulmonary metastases, the tumor was injected intravenously and from 3 to 10 days later, therapy was instituted.[38-40] An illustration of the phenomenon is presented in Table 2 using the NK-resistant, B16 melanoma.[43-44] In this particular experiment, mice bearing established pulmonary micrometastases 3 days after the i.v. injection of B16 melanoma cells received the adoptive transfer of LAK cells on days 3 and 6. Mice also received i.p. injections of Hank's Balanced Salt Solution (HBSS) or recombinant IL-2 (RIL-2) at a dose of 6000 units per injection three times a day from days 3 through 8. Numerous micrometastatic foci were evident histologically when the immunotherapy was begun. The mice were ear-tagged, randomized, and the number of pulmonary nodules evaluated in a blinded fashion 14 days after tumor injection. Administration of LAK cells

Table 3
LAK CELLS PLUS RECOMBINANT IL-2 MARKEDLY REDUCE THE NUMBER OF ARTIFICIALLY INDUCED, ESTABLISHED PULMONARY METASTASES OF MCA-105 SARCOMA

Treatment group[a]	No. of metastases per mouse[b]	Mean	p[c]
HBSS	250,250,178,158,141,134,114,98,77,0	140	—
RIL-2	250,250,250,222,163,68	201	0.16
LAK + HBSS	202,115,102,84,21,2	88	0.26
LAK + RIL-2	31,6,1,0,0,0	6	0.01

[a] The number of MCA-105 sarcoma cells injected i.v. was 3×10^5. RIL-2 (7,500 units per injection) or HBSS was injected intraperitoneally approximately every 8 hr from days 3 through 5 after tumor injection; 1×10^8 LAK cells were injected i.v. on day 3. LAK cells were generated by the incubation of fresh splenocytes in CM containing pure recombinant IL-2 for 3 days in vitro.

[b] No. of metastases at day 13.

[c] Wilcoxon rank sum test of treated groups compared to group receiving HBSS alone (two-sided).

From Mulé, J. J. et al., *Cancer Res.*, 46, 676, 1985. With permission.

alone or RIL-2 alone slightly reduced the number of metastases (mean = 126 and 121, respectively). These slight reductions are often seen in our experiments, but they are rarely statistically significant due to variation within each treated group. However, mice given LAK cells plus RIL-2 had an average of 12 metastases, a reduction in pulmonary B16 melanoma metastases of 93%. A similar therapy experiment using the NK-resistant, weakly immunogenic MCA-105 sarcoma is shown in Table 3.[43] The combination of LAK cells plus RIL-2 effectively reduced the number of established metastatic foci by 96%. As shown in Table 4, reduction of metastases was dependent on the transfer of LAK cells since fresh, normal splenocytes, splenocytes cultured for 3 days without RIL-2 or either combined with RIL-2 failed to mediate any significant antitumor effect upon adoptive transfer.[39] The appearance of the lungs from a representative experiment is shown in Figure 1. Thus, the adoptive transfer of LAK cells plus repetitive injections of recombinant IL-2 was necessary in these models to mediate antitumor effects.

The time course of LAK cell activation required in vitro before adoptive transfer of these cells is shown in Table 5.[39] LAK cells were generated in vitro from normal C57BL/6 splenocytes cultured in RIL-2 for 1 to 4 days before i.v. infusion into mice bearing established, 3 day MCA-105 pulmonary metastases. RIL-2 was administered concomitantly and at 14 or 15 days the number of pulmonary metastases was evaluated. In both experiments shown, splenocytes incubated in RIL-2 for 3 days were most effective in reducing the number of tumor nodules upon adoptive transfer. The antitumor efficacy of LAK cells plus RIL-2 on established 3-day pulmonary metastases is highly reproducible. Figure 2 shows a compendium of 44 consecutive experiments evaluating LAK cells plus varying doses of systematically administered RIL-2 on the percent reduction of metastatic nodules. By titration analysis, it is clear that reduction in metastases was most pronounced with the higher doses of RIL-2 administered intraperitoneally. As will be discussed later, elevating the dose of RIL-2 to 100,000 units per injection can dramatically reduce pulmonary sarcoma metastases when used alone. The successful therapy of pulmonary metastases has been seen not only when using the weakly immunogenic MCA-105 tumor but for the treatment of two nonimmunogenic

Table 4
IMMUNOTHERAPEUTIC EFFECT OF LAK CELLS AND RECOMBINANT IL-2 ON ESTABLISHED PULMONARY SARCOMA METASTASES

Cells[b]	No. of metastases (mean) at day 13[a]	
	HBSS	RIL-2
None	228	152
Cultured splenocytes	183	156
Fresh splenocytes	214	191
LAK	200	20[c]

[a] The number of MCA sarcoma cells injected intravenously was 3×10^5; each group contained 6 mice. RIL-2 (15,000 units per injection) or HBSS was injected intraperitoneally approximately every 8 hr from days 3 through 8 after tumor injection.

[b] 1×10^8 LAK cells, fresh normal splenocytes, or normal splenocytes cultured for 3 days without RIL-2 were injected intravenously on days 3 and 6 after tumor injection.

[c] LAK + RIL-2 vs. RIL-2 alone; $p < 0.01$.[39]

From Mulé, J. J. et al., *J. Immunol.*, 135, 646, 1985. With permission.

methylcholanthrene-induced sarcomas, MCA-101 and MCA-102, as well as in the treatment of pulmonary metastases from the MCA-38 adenocarcinoma, the B16 melanoma and the M-3 melanoma in C3H mice.

Since previous work from our laboratory has shown that LAK cells allogeneic to fresh, tumor targets are equally lytic as syngeneic LAK cells in short-term, ^{51}Cr-release assays,[25,28] we analyzed the antitumor efficacy of allogeneic LAK cells in vivo. In the three separate experiments shown in Table 6, LAK cells generated from DBA/2 (H-2^d) splenocytes were as effective in reducing established 3-day pulmonary metastases of MCA-105 sarcoma when combined with RIL-2 (mean = 22, 20, and 50 in Experiments 1, 2, and 3, respectively) as those generated from syngeneic, B6 splenocytes (mean = 21, 4, and 48 in Experiments 1, 2, and 3, respectively) when compared to HBSS alone (mean = 138, 111, and 225 in Experiments 1, 2, and 3, respectively). Both allogeneic and syngeneic LAK cells displayed similar lytic capacity in vitro (see legend to Table 5). Thus, although restriction at murine major histocompatibility loci has been shown to be necessary in the successful adoptive immunotherapy of certain tumors when using specifically sensitized immune cells,[45] this phenomenon is not a requirement in the treatment of metastases by LAK cells. The evidence presented that allogeneic LAK cells have antimetastatic capacity upon adoptive transfer, combined with the fact that they are dependent on IL-2 for survival, provides the possibility for their use in a clinical setting.

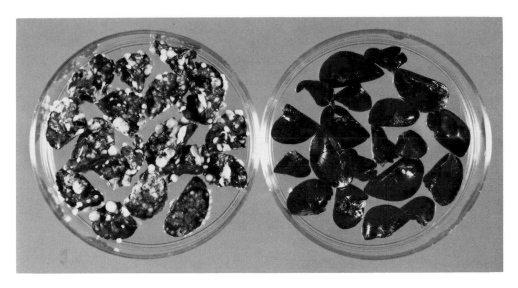

FIGURE 1. Representative lungs of four mice from group given HBSS (left) or LAK cells plus RIL-2 (right). (From Mulé, J. J. et al., *Science,* 225, 1487, 1984. With permission.)

Table 5
KINETICS OF LAK CELL GENERATION IN VITRO VS. CAPACITY TO REDUCE ESTABLISHED PULMONARY SARCOMA METASTASES IN VIVO[a]

| | | No. of metastases (mean)[d] | |
Group	Treatment[b]	Experiment 1	Experiment 2
A	HBSS	250	250
B	RIL-2	199	250
C	Day 1 LAK[c] + RIL-2	223	205
D	Day 2 LAK + RIL-2	80	250
E	Day 3 LAK + RIL-2	11	21
F	Day 4 LAK + RIL-2	42	90

[a] The number of MCA sarcoma cells injected intravenously was 3 × 10^5; groups contained 5 to 8 mice. Lungs were removed 15 and 14 days after tumor injection in Experiments 1 and 2, respectively.

[b] RIL-2 or HBSS was injected intraperitoneally approximately every 8 hr from days 3 through 8. Mice received 25,000 units per injection or 20,000 units per injection of RIL-2 in Experiments 1 and 2, respectively.

[c] 1 × 10^8 LAK cells were injected intravenously on days 3 and 6 after tumor injection. LAK cells were generated in vitro from normal splenocytes cultured in RIL-2 for 1, 2, 3, or 4 days before infusion.

[d] Statistical significance of differences: Experiment 1 = A vs.: B, NS; C, NS; D, <0.01; E, p<0.005; F, <0.01. E vs.: C, <0.01; D, <0.01; F, <0.02. Experiment 2 = A vs.: B, NS; C, NS; D, NS; E, <0.001; F, <0.03. E vs.: C, <0.01; D, <0.01; F, <0.02.

From Mulé, J. J. et al., *J. Immunol.,* 135, 646, 1985. With permission.

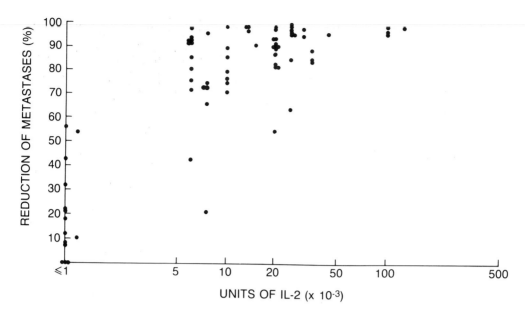

FIGURE 2.   Reduction of established 3-day pulmonary sarcoma metastases by LAK cells plus RIL-2 in 44 consecutive experiments. Each dot represents a separate experimental determination in which mice receiving LAK cells plus RIL-2 were compared to mice treated with HBSS alone. Therapy with LAK cells plus RIL-2 was initiated 3-days after the i.v. injection of MCA-induced sarcoma cells. RIL-2 was administered intraperitoneally approximately every 8 hr for 5 days. Increasing doses of RIL-2 led to increasing reduction in the number of pulmonary metastases when 1×10^8 LAK cells were administered intravenously concurrently on day 3 or on days 3 and 6. (From Mulé, J. J. et al., *J. Immunol.*, 136, 3899, 1986. With permission.)

Table 6
ALLOGENEIC LAK CELLS ARE EFFECTIVE IN REDUCING THE NUMBERS OF ESTABLISHED 3-DAY MCA-105 PULMONARY MICROMETASTASES UPON ADOPTIVE TRANSFER

| | Days after | | | No. of metastases (mean)[d] | |
| | tumor | (A) | (B) | (C) | (D) |
Experiment[a]	injection	HBSS	RIL-2[b]	Syngeneic (B6) LAK + RIL-2[c]	Allogeneic (DBA) LAK + RIL-2
1	13	138	75	21	22
2	15	111	—	4	20
3	15	225	117	48	50

[a]   The number of MCA sarcoma cells injected intravenously was 3×10^5 in Experiments 1 and 3, and 2×10^5 in Experiment 2. Groups contained between 5 and 10 animals.

[b]   RIL-2 was injected intraperitoneally approximately every 8 hr from days 3 through 8 after tumor injection; mice received 34,000 units per injection in Experiment 1 and 42,500 units per injection in Experiments 2 and 3.

[c]   The number of LAK cells injected intravenously on day 3 and 6 was 5×10^7 in Experiments 1 and 3, and 1×10^8 in Experiment 2. The specific cytotoxicity in vitro at an effector:target cell ratio of 100:1 was: in Experiment 1, 57 ± 4 and 64 ± 2 (for the day 3 and day 6 injection, respectively) for B6 LAK cells vs. 55 ± 6 and 51 ± 2 for DBA LAK cells; in Experiment 2, 40 ± 6 and 33 ± 3 (for the day 3 and day 6 injection, respectively) for B6 LAK cells vs. 35 ± 4 and 30 ± 4 for DBA LAK cells; in Experiment 3, 22 ± 2 and 40 ± 2 (for the day 3 and day 6 injection, respectively) for B6 LAK cells vs. 20 ± 5 and 58 ± 9 for DBA LAK cells.

[d]   Statistical significance of differences: Experiment 1. A vs.: B, NS; C, $p < 0.005$; D, $p < 0.01$. B vs.: C, $p < 0.05$; D, $p < 0.02$. C vs.: D, NS. Experiment 2. A vs.: C, $p < 0.005$; D, $p < 0.005$. C vs.: D, $p < 0.02$. Experiment 3. A vs.: B, NS; C, $p < 0.005$; D, $p < 0.005$. B vs.: C, NS; D, NS. C vs.: D, NS.

From Mulé, J. J. et al., *J. Immunol.*, 135, 646, 1985. With permission.

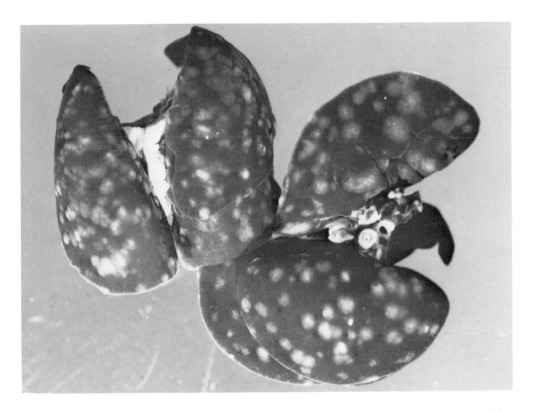

FIGURE 3. Representative lungs of 2 mice in which multiple sarcoma macrometastases are clearly evident on the lung surfaces at day 10 after i.v. injection of MCA-105. Therapy was begun with LAK cells and RIL-2 at this stage of metastatic tumor development. (From Mulé, J. J. et al., *J. Immunol.*, 135, 646, 1985. With permission.)

We have also tested the efficacy of the combined therapy of LAK cells and RIL-2 on pulmonary macrometastases established in the lung 10 days after the i.v. injection of MCA-105 sarcoma cells.[39] Figure 3 shows the stage of metastatic development when treatment was begun; numerous distinct foci of tumor were evident on the lung surface. A representative experiment illustrating the effectiveness of LAK cells plus RIL-2 therapy in the treatment of these larger metastases is seen in Table 7. Note that there was a reduction in pulmonary metastases when RIL-2 was administered alone, which is commonly seen when higher doses of RIL-2 are used in this day 10 treatment model. However, when LAK cells were given in conjunction with RIL-2 a more marked reduction in the number of pulmonary metastases was obtained (from 227 metastases in control mice to an average of 6 metastases in animals treated with LAK cells plus 20,000 units of recombinant IL-2 three times a day). Figure 4 shows a compendium of six consecutive experiments in which escalating doses of systemically administered RIL-2 combined with LAK cells was highly effective in reducing sarcoma macrometastases.

III. THE COMBINATION OF LYMPHOKINE-ACTIVATED KILLER CELLS AND RECOMBINANT IL-2 MARKEDLY REDUCES ESTABLISHED LIVER METASTASES

In a new experimental model designed to produce metastases solely in the liver, Lafreniere and Rosenberg undertook studies to assess the effectiveness of adoptive therapy with RIL-2 alone and LAK cells plus RIL-2 on metastatic foci in this location.

Table 7
TREATMENT OF ESTABLISHED (DAY 10) PULMONARY METASTASES WITH LAK CELLS

Recombinant IL-2 (units)[a]	(Mean number of metastases)	
	No LAK cells	Plus LAK cells[b]
0	227	210
1,000	208	192
6,000	171	61 ($p<0.05$)
20,000	56 ($p<0.05$)	6 ($p<0.02$)

[a] IL-2 injected intraperitoneally every 8 hr from days 10 through 17.
[b] 10^8 LAK cells injected intravenously on days 10 and 13 after tumor injection.

From Mule, J. J. et al., *J. Immunol.*, 135, 646, 1985. With permission.

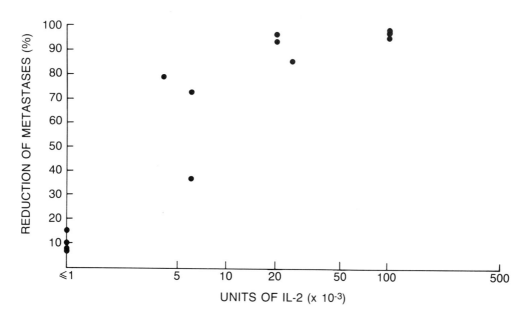

FIGURE 4.   Reduction of established 10-day pulmonary sarcoma metastases by LAK cells plus RIL-2 in 6 consecutive experiments. Each dot represents a separate experimental determination in which mice receiving LAK cells plus RIL-2 were compared to mice treated with HBSS alone. Therapy with LAK cells plus RIL-2 was initiated 10 days after the i.v. injection of MCA-105 sarcoma cells. RIL-2 was administered intraperitoneally approximately every 8 hr for 5 days. Increasing doses of RIL-2 led to increasing reduction in the number of pulmonary metastases when 1×10^8 LAK cells were administered intravenously concurrently on days 10 and 13.

This model also tested the ability of intravenously injected LAK cells to mediate antitumor effects in an organ that did not represent the first capillary bed, (i.e., the lung) encountered by LAK cells after i.v. injection.[41,42] The selective induction of hepatic metastases is based on the injection of tumor cells into the spleen followed by immediate splenectomy. Tumor cells flow out the splenic vein into the portal vein and lodge in the liver where established metastases are formed. A typical experiment in which 3-day established MCA-105 sarcoma hepatic metastases were treated with increasing

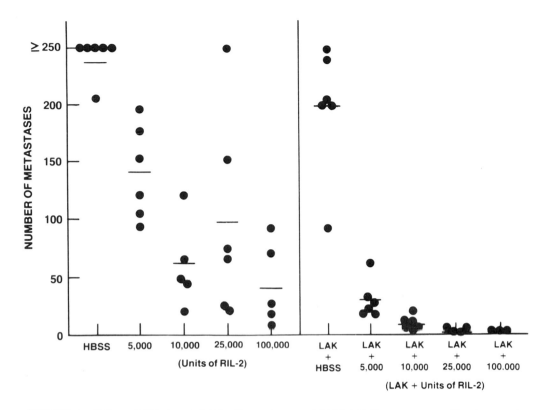

FIGURE 5.   Effect of RIL-2 and LAK cells on therapy of MCA-105 liver metastases. The decrease in experimentally induced MCA 105 liver metastases caused by injection of RIL-2 given intraperitoneally every 8 hr (left), was compared to the same doses of RIL-2 administered concomitantly with 1×10^8 syngeneic LAK cells generated in vitro. RIL-2 was given intraperitoneally beginning on day 3 and LAK cells were given intravenously at day 3 and 6 posttumor injection (right). The number of metastases were counted in a coded fashion at day 14 after MCA-105 injection. Each dot represents a measure of the number of liver metastases in an individual mouse. (From Lafreniere, R. and Rosenberg, S. A., *Cancer Res.*, 45, 3735, 1985. With permission.)

doses of RIL-2 with or without LAK cells is shown in Figure 5. Note that higher doses of RIL-2 alone have a small effect in reducing the number of hepatic metastases but a very dramatic effect is seen when LAK cells are added to this IL-2 therapy. This experiment also serves to illustrate the variation seen in this in vivo therapeutic assay. The successful therapy of established hepatic metastases with LAK cells plus RIL-2 is highly reproducible and has been seen in 16 consecutive experiments with the weakly immunogenic MCA-105 sarcoma (Figure 6) as well as in experiments with the nonimmunogenic MCA-102 sarcoma and the MCA-38 adenocarcinoma (Figure 7).[42]

LAK cells are larger than resting lymphocytes and the possibility existed that many would lodge in the lung and thus would not circulate to the liver in amounts sufficient enough to mediate the most optimal antitumor effect given the number of LAK cells administered. Thus, a method was developed for the injection of LAK cells directly into the portal vein of the anesthetized mouse and i.p. administration of RIL-2 was then begun shortly thereafter. LAK cells administered intraportally were able to mediate better antitumor activity against the MCA-105 sarcoma compared to the same number of LAK cells given i.v. in the lateral tail vein, presumably due to the larger number of LAK cells that reach the liver when injected intraportally.[42]

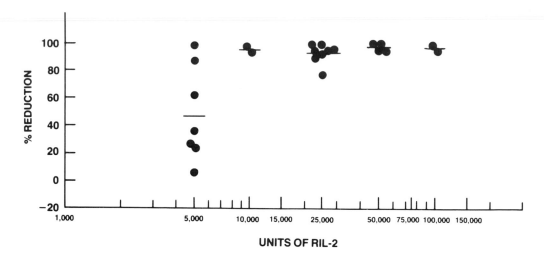

FIGURE 6.   Effect of LAK cells plus increasing doses of RIL-2 on MCA-105 liver metastases in 16 consecutive experiments. Each dot represents a separate experimental determination. Each animal was injected with 3×10^5 MCA-105 cells and treated starting on day 3 with RIL-2, i.p. every 8 hr. Increasing doses of RIL-2 led to increasing reduction in the number of hepatic metastases when 1×10^8 LAK cells were administered intravenously concurrently on day 3 and day 6. (From Lafreniere, R. and Rosenberg, S. A., *Cancer Res.*, 45, 3735, 1985. With permission.)

IV. REGRESSION OF ESTABLISHED PULMONARY AND HEPATIC METASTASES MEDIATED BY THE SYSTEMIC ADMINISTRATION OF HIGH-DOSE RECOMBINANT IL-2

Because recombinant IL-2 is capable of efficiently generating LAK cells in vitro, and because the systemic administration of LAK cells has potent antitumor activities, we studied the possible use of high-dose recombinant IL-2 administered directly to tumor-bearing mice, aiming to generate LAK cells in vivo and mediate tumor regression. Initial experiments in our laboratory by Chang et al.,[46] in which mice received continuous infusions of recombinant IL-2 either intraperitoneally or subcutaneously, using an osmotic pump, indicated that LAK cells could be generated in the spleens of mice in vivo. To further test the ability of RIL-2 to induce LAK cell activity in vivo, mice were injected intraperitoneally with varying doses of RIL-2 approximately every 8 hr for 5 days. On the morning of day 6, mice were killed and LAK activity in spleens was assessed using fresh MCA sarcoma target cells. As shown in Table 8, increasing doses of RIL-2 resulted in a successive increase in the lytic activity in the spleen against fresh sarcoma cells.

C57BL/6 mice bearing established 3-day pulmonary micrometastases of the MCA-105 sarcoma were treated with varying doses of RIL-2 administered intraperitoneally every 8 hr for 5 days. The number of pulmonary metastases was evaluated at 15 days. A representative experiment is shown in Figure 8. Each dot represents the measurement of a single mouse. Recombinant IL-2 at a dose of 50,000 or 100,000 units was capable of significantly reducing the number of pulmonary metastases. Mice receiving either HBSS alone, or 5,000 or 20,000 units of IL-2 had a mean number of metastases of >250, 212, and 214, respectively (no significant difference between these groups). Mice receiving 50,000 or 100,000 units of IL-2 experienced a marked reduction of metastases with a mean of 19 and 61 respectively ($p = 0.002$ and $p = 0.003$, respectively, compared to HBSS group). Figure 9 shows the reproducibility of this phenomenon in 36 consecutive experiments. The percent reduction in 3-day pulmonary metastases of mice treated with RIL-2 at three dosage ranges is compared to mice treated with HBSS

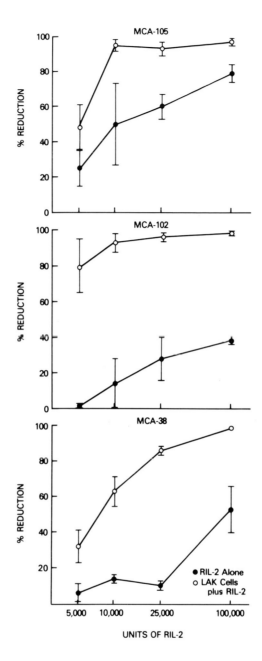

FIGURE 7.   Dose titration of RIL-2 and effects of LAK cells plus increasing doses of RIL-2 on experimentally induced hepatic metastases from multiple murine tumors. The effects of increasing doses of RIL-2 against hepatic metastases are demonstrated for two murine sarcomas (MCA-105 and MCA-102) and one murine adenocarcinoma (MCA-38). Increasing doses of RIL-2 led to increasing reduction in the number of hepatic metastases (●—●). When 1 × 10⁸ syngeneic LAK cells were systemically administered intravenously on days 3 and 6 with the same doses of RIL-2 (●—●) the percent reduction in liver metastases was significantly increased over that observed with RIL-2 alone. Each measure reflects the mean percent reduction ± SEM for all experiments performed (MCA-105 RIL-2 alone, 20 consecutive experiments; LAK plus RIL-2, 16 consecutive experiments; MCA-102 RIL-2 alone, 2 consecutive experiments; LAK plus RIL-2, 2 consecutive experiments; MCA-38, RIL-2 alone, 2 consecutive experiments; LAK plus RIL-2, 2 consecutive experiments. (From Lafreniere, R. and Rosenberg, S. A., *J. Immunol.*, 135, 4273, 1985. With permission.)

Table 8

INDUCTION OF LAK ACTIVITY IN SPLEENS OF MICE TREATED WITH RECOMBINANT IL-2

IL-2[a] (units)	Lytic activity vs. MCA-102 E:T,[b] %[c]	
	100:1	20:1
0	−1 ± 2	−3 ± 3
75,000	14 ± 1	−2 ± 1
100,000	17 ± 2	1 ± 2
150,000	19 ± 1	9 ± 1
200,000	21 ± 4	11 ± 1
400,000	32 ± 2	16 ± 4

[a] IL-2 was administered for 5 days intraperitoneally in 0.5 mℓ, approximately every 8 hr.

[b] Effector to target ratio in 4-hr, chromium-51 release assay.

[c] Percent lysis ± SEM.

From Rosenberg, S. A. et al., *J. Exp. Med.,* 161, 1169, 1985. With permission.

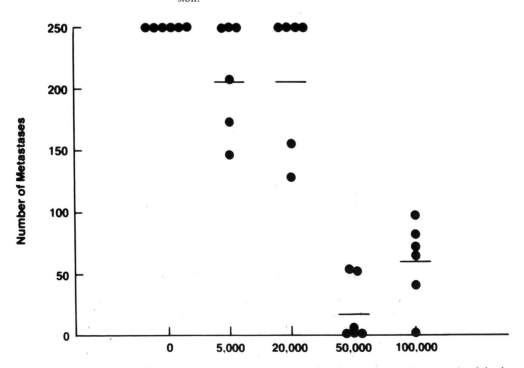

FIGURE 8.   Treatment of day 3 pulmonary metastases with recombinant IL-2. 3 days after i.v. injection of 3 × 10⁵ sarcoma cells, mice began therapy with varying doses of recombinant IL-2 administered intraperitoneally three times daily for 5 days. At day 15, mice were killed and the number of pulmonary nodules was determined. Each dot represents the measurement of a single mouse. Doses of 50,000 to 100,000 units IL-2 administered in this schedule significantly reduced the number of pulmonary metastases compared to mice receiving no IL-2 ($p = 0.002$ and $p = 0.003$, respectively). (From Rosenberg, S. A. et al., *J. Exp. Med.,* 161, 1169, 1985. With permission.)

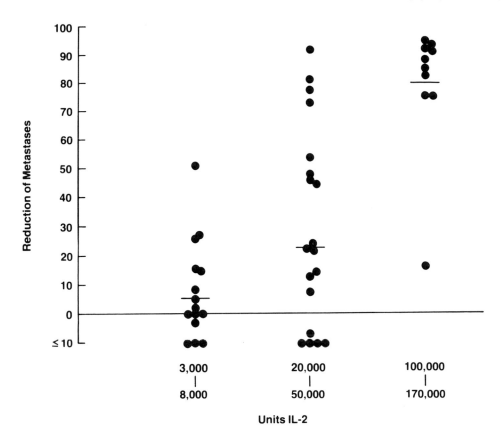

FIGURE 9. Results of 36 consecutive experiments evaluating the ability of varying doses of recombinant IL-2 to reduce day 3 pulmonary metastases. Each dot represents a separate experimental measurement in which mice receiving IL-2 were compared to mice treated with HBSS alone. Therapy with varying doses of IL-2 was initiated 3 days after the i.v. injection of MCA-105 sarcoma cells. IL-2 was administered intraperitoneally approximately every 8 hr for 5 days. Doses of 100,000 to 170,000 units IL-2 significantly reduced pulmonary metastases in 9 of 10 experiments. (From Rosenberg, S. A. et al., *J. Exp. Med.*, 161, 1169, 1985. With permission.)

alone. Mice receiving between 3000 and 8000 units of RIL-2 had 5.7 ± 5.0% (mean ± SE) reductions in pulmonary metastases, mice receiving 20,000 to 50,000 units of RIL-2 had 22.2 ± 9.2% reductions, and mice receiving 100,000 to 170,000 units IL-2 experienced 79.5 ± 7.3% reductions in pulmonary metastases. The dosage range of 20,000 to 50,000 units RIL-2 appeared to be on the threshold of mediating antitumor effects, and although significant variation was seen in different experiments at this dose range, the use of 100,000 units or more consistently reduced pulmonary metastases in nine of ten experiments. Figure 10 shows that the systemic administration of high-dose RIL-2 was also effective against pulmonary metastases of the MCA-106 sarcoma and the B16 melanoma.

The antitumor efficacy of systemically administered high-dose RIL-2 has recently been evaluated on 3-day established hepatic metastases of the MCA-105 sarcoma. Results of 42 determinations from 20 consecutive experiments are shown in Figure 11.[47] The reduction in metastases was variable at RIL-2 doses less than or equal to 25,000 units with a percent reduction ranging from 0 to 97% (mean 42% in 28 determinations). At doses from 1000 to 5000, 10,000 to 15,000 units, and 25,000 units the percent reduction over HBSS was statistically significant ($p < 0.05$) in 2/12, 2/4, and 8/12 determinations respectively. At doses greater than 25,000 units, the reduction in liver

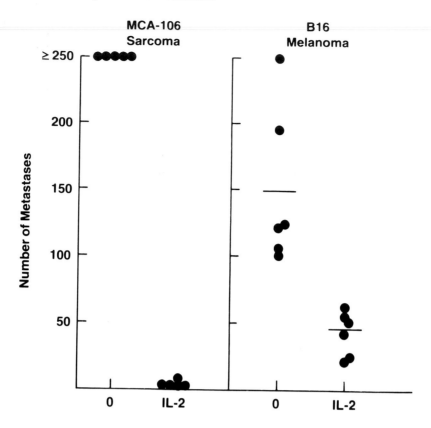

FIGURE 10.   Reduction of pulmonary metastases of the MCA-106 sarcoma (left) and the B16 melanoma (right) by administration of recombinant IL-2. 3 days after i.v. injection of either MCA-106 sarcoma or B16 melanoma cells, therapy was initiated with 100,000 units recombinant IL-2 given intraperitoneally approximately every 8 hr for 5 days. On day 15, mice were killed and pulmonary nodules were counted. Each dot represents the measurement of a single mouse. A significant reduction in the number of pulmonary metastases was seen in the treatment of both tumors when IL-2 was administered ($p = 0.006$ for the MCA-106 sarcoma, and $p = 0.005$ for the B16 melanoma). (From Rosenberg, S. A. et al., *J. Exp. Med.*, 161, 1169, 1985. With permission.)

metastases was highly reproducible with a range of percent reduction of 66 to 95% (mean 83% in 14 determinations); 14/14 determinations had a statistically significant decrease in the number of metastases ($p < 0.0005$). At doses equal to or greater than 100,000 units given i.p. approximately every 8 hr, significant toxicity was seen by 5 days that limited the amount of RIL-2 that could be given in any one experiment.

Since the combination of LAK cells plus relatively low doses of recombinant IL-2 markedly reduced 10-day pulmonary macrometastases, we tested the antitumor efficacy of high doses of RIL-2 alone administered systemically. Mice bearing 10-day pulmonary sarcoma nodules received RIL-2 three times a day for 5 days. In these experiments, mice were usually killed on the 18th day after tumor cell injection, and the number of pulmonary metastases was determined in a blinded fashion. Figure 12 shows 15 consecutive experiments evaluating the efficacy of treatment with varying doses of RIL-2 alone.[48] Doses at 0 to 6000 units RIL-2 reduced the number of pulmonary nodules by 34.6 ± 13.3%; 20,000 to 50,000 units RIL-2 reduced 10-day pulmonary metastases by 89.4 ± 3.4%, and 100,000 to 200,000 units RIL-2 reduced pulmonary metastases by 79.6 ± 4.7%. A comparison of results using RIL-2 alone to treat 3-day (Figure 9) and 10-day (Figure 12) pulmonary metastases suggested that lower doses of RIL-2

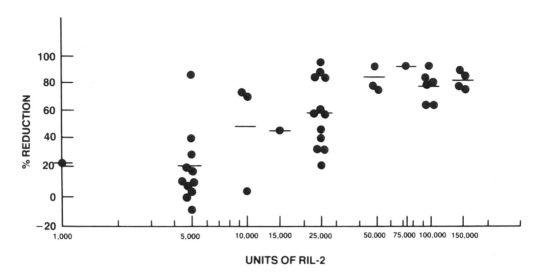

FIGURE 11.   Dose titration of the ability of RIL-2 to reduce liver metastases in 20 consecutive experiments. Each dot represents a separate experimental determination. Each animal was injected with 3×10^5 MCA-105 cells and treated on day 3 with RIL-2, i.p. every 8 hr. Increasing doses of RIL-2 led to increasing reduction in the number of hepatic metastases. (From Lafreniere, R. and Rosenberg, S. A., *J. Immunol.*, 45, 3735, 1985. With permission.)

were more effective against day 10 tumors than against day-3 tumors. Two experiments designed to test this observation directly are presented in Table 9. The MCA-105 tumor was injected intravenously on day 0, and beginning either 3 or 10 days later, therapy with RIL-2 was initiated for 5 days. All mice were killed on day 15, and the number of pulmonary tumors was determined. In experiment 1 (Table 9), control mice (HBSS alone) had a mean of 56 metastases compared to a mean of 47 metastases in mice that started RIL-2 treatment at 6000 units three times daily on day 3, and 8 metastases in mice that started RIL-2 treatment on day 10. Similarly, in experiment 2, control mice had a mean of 45 metastases compared to 54 metastases in mice starting treatment with 20,000 units IL-2 three times daily on day 3, and 6 metastases in mice starting treatment on day 10. These experiments demonstrated that day-10 metastases from the MCA-105 sarcoma were more susceptible to RIL-2 therapy than were day-3 metastases. The greater sensitivity of 10 day tumors to RIL-2 therapy may reflect the state of activation of the hosts' immune system which is then augmented by the administration of RIL-2.

V. POSSIBLE MECHANISMS OF ADOPTIVE IMMUNOTHERAPY WITH LYMPHOKINE-ACTIVATED KILLER CELLS AND RECOMBINANT IL-2

We have been investigating the mechanisms of action of tumor destruction in vivo by LAK cells plus RIL-2. We have examined whether or not the host contributes a necessary component to the adoptive immunotherapy by using recipient mice bearing 3-day pulmonary or hepatic metastases that have been immunosuppressed. Mice received 500 rad total body irradiation 1 to 6 hr before the injection of tumor cells and therapy was begun 3 days later.[39] A dose of 20,000 to 100,000 units of RIL-2 were given intraperitoneally every 8 hr for 5 days beginning on day 3. On days 3 and 6, 1×10^8 syngeneic LAK cells were given intravenously. Mice were sacrificed at 2 weeks and the numbers of lung (Table 10) and liver (Figure 13) metastases were evaluated. Results in Table 10 and Figure 13 show that the combination of LAK cells plus RIL-2 effectively reduce metastases in both normal and irradiated mice. In contrast, although high

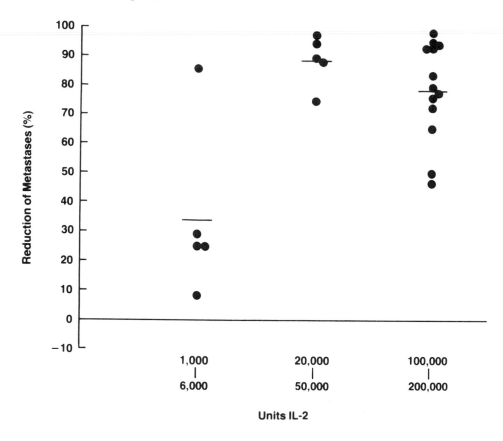

FIGURE 12.   Results of 15 consecutive experiments evaluating the ability of treatment with recombinant IL-2 to reduce the number of 10-day pulmonary metastases. Each dot represents a separate experimental measurement in which mice receiving IL-2 were compared to mice treated with HBSS alone. Therapy was initiated with varying doses of recombinant IL-2 given intraperitoneally approximately every 8 hr for 5 days 10 days after i.v. injection of MCA-105 sarcoma cells. On days 15 to 18, mice were killed and pulmonary metastases were counted. Doses > 20,000 units administered on this schedule were consistently able to reduce the number of pulmonary metastases compared to that of control mice. (From Rosenberg, S. A. et al., *J. Exp. Med.,* 161, 1169, 1985. With permission.)

doses of RIL-2 alone (50,000 to 100,000 units) can reduce the number of pulmonary and hepatic metastases in normal mice, this antitumor effect is completely lost in the irradiated mice. Similarly, we have found that LAK cells plus RIL-2, but not RIL-2 alone, effectively reduce established pulmonary metastases in mice that are T-cell depleted (''B'' mice) by the combination of adult thymectomy and lethal irradiation followed by reconstitution with T-cell depleted bone marrow cells (Table 11). These findings suggest that LAK cells do not require a fully competent or intact immune system to mediate antitumor effects in vivo. However, we have not defined whether the host contributes a relatively radio-resistant component to the response. Of clinical relevance is the fact that cancer patients immunosuppressed by chemotherapy or radiotherapy can potentially serve as candidates for immunotherapy using LAK cells and recombinant IL-2.

Exposure of LAK cells to 3000 rad of irradiation reduces the capacity of these cells to eliminate established pulmonary metastases upon i.v. transfer when combined with RIL-2 (Table 12).[39] Since we have found that irradiated LAK cells retain lytic activity in vitro in 4 hr ^{51}Cr-release assays, the loss of antitumor activity in vivo probably reflects a requirement for proliferation and expansion of these cells in the presence of

Table 9

TREATMENT OF ESTABLISHED
(DAY 3 AND 10) PULMONARY
METASTASES WITH
RECOMBINANT IL-2

RIL-2[a] (units)	Begin treatment on: (mean number of metastases)	
	day 3	day 10
Experiment 1:		
0	56	—
6,000	47	8
	($p = 0.23$)[b]	($p = 0.02$)
Experiment 2:		
0	45	—
20,000	54	6
	($p = 0.79$)	($p = 0.006$)

[a] IL-2 was administered intraperitoneally in 0.5 mℓ three times a day for 5 days starting either 3 days or 10 days after tumor injection.
[b] Wilcoxon rank sum test comparing group receiving IL-2 to group receiving no IL-2 (two-sided).

From Rosenberg, S. A. et al., *J. Exp. Med.*, 161, 1169, 1985. With permission.

Table 10

TREATMENT OF ESTABLISHED
PULMONARY METASTASES (DAY 3)
WITH RIL-2: EFFECT OF HOST
IRRADIATION

R-IL-2[a]	Normal Mice[d]		Irradiated Mice[b,d]	
	No LAK	+ LAK[c]	No LAK	+ LAK[c]
0	>250	Nd	>250	Nd
20,000	214 ± 23	19 ± 5	>250	44 ± 22
100,000	61 ± 14	11 ± 5	>250	67 ± 15

[a] Intraperitoneally, every 8 hr from days 3 to 8.
[b] 500 rad total body irradiation.
[c] 10^8 LAK cells given intravenously on day 3 and day 6.
[d] No. of metastases.

From Rosenberg, S. A. and Mulé, J. J., *Surgery*, 98, 437, 1985. With permission.

RIL-2. To examine this point, Ettinghausen et al. have used a technique that involves the labeling of dividing cells in vivo by the injection of 5-[^{125}I]-iodo-2-deoxyuridine (^{125}I-UdR).[49,50] Mice were treated with either HBSS (controls), LAK cells, RIL-2, or LAK cells plus RIL-2 and ^{125}I-UdR incorporation into various organs was assessed. A single i.v. injection of 1×10^8 LAK cells was given on day 0 and either 6000 units of RIL-2 or an equivalent volume of HBSS was i.p. injected 3 times a day for 7 days. The raw data and calculated proliferation index for ^{125}IUdR incorporation into lungs, liver,

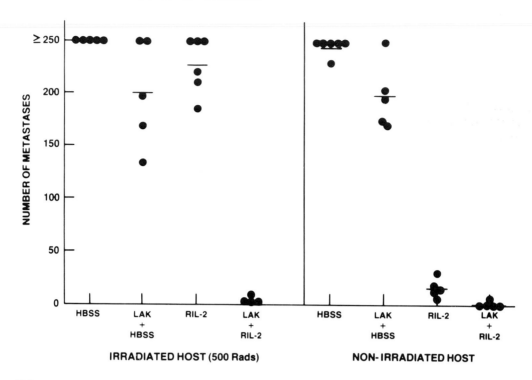

FIGURE 13.   Effect of host irradiation on RIL-2 and LAK + RIL-2 therapy of liver metastases. At day 0, one half of mice were given a sublethal total body irradiation dose of 500 rad with Cesium-[137]; 1 hr later they were anesthetized and injected intrasplenically with 3×10^5 MCA-105 cells (left). 50,000 units of RIL-2 were given intraperitoneally every 8 hr for 5 days beginning on day 3. 1×10^8 syngeneic LAK cells were given i.v. on day 3 and 6. Mice were ear-tagged and sacrificed at day 14 and liver metastases were counted blindly. High doses of RIL-2 alone could reduce the number of liver metastases in the normal but not in the irradiated mice. LAK cells plus RIL-2 effectively reduced metastases in both normal and irradiated mice. (From Lafreniere, R. and Rosenberg, S. A., *Cancer Res.*, 45, 3735, 1985. With permission.)

Table 11

LAK CELLS PLUS RIL-2, BUT NOT RIL-2 ALONE, REDUCES ESTABLISHED MCA-105 PULMONARY METASTASES IN T-CELL DEPLETED MICE

Experiment No[a]	Group	Normal mice			"B" mice[b]		
		No. of metastases[c]	Mean	p[d]	No. of metastases	Mean	p
1	HBSS	250,250,250,250,250,250	250	—	250,250,250,250,250	250	—
	RIL-2	250,46,31,11,9,3	58	0.02	250,250,250,194,178	224	0.3
2	HBSS	155,131,127,123,16	110	—	250,250,193,191,154	208	—
	RIL-2	59,41,31,16,5	30	0.06	236,232,107,92	167	0.33
	LAK cells + RIL-2	16,4,1,1,0	4	0.01	35,6,1,0,0	8	0.01

[a]   Treatment of established 10-day and 3-day pulmonary metastases in experiments 1 and 2, respectively. 100,000 and 10,000 Units of RIL-2 were given three times a day intraperitoneally for 5 days in experiments 1 and 2, respectively.

[b]   Adult mice were thymectomized and total body irradiated 2 weeks later with 900 rad. The mice received 3×10^6 bone marrow cells intravenously that were depleted of T-cells with monoclonal antibody and complement 1 to 2 hr later.

[c]   At day 17 and 14, respectively in experiments 1 and 2.

[d]   Wilcoxon rank sum test of treated groups compared to group receiving HBSS alone (two-sided).

From Mulé, J. J. et al., *J. Immunol.*, 136, 3899, 1986. With permission.

Table 12
IRRADIATED LAK CELLS HAVE A REDUCED CAPACITY TO IMPACT ON ESTABLISHED 3-DAY MCA-105 PULMONARY MICROMETASTASES UPON ADOPTIVE TRANSFER

		No. of metastases (mean)[d]				
Experiment[a]	Days after tumor injection	(A) HBSS	(B) RIL-2[b]	(C) LAK + HBSS	(D) LAK + RIL-2	(E) Irradiated LAK[c] + RIL-2
1	15	250	250	250	62	238
2	14	151	—	—	11	95
3	13	214	186	—	4	113

[a] The number of MCA sarcoma cells injected intravenously was 3×10^5 in Experiment 1 and 3, and 2×10^5 in Experiment 2. Experiments 1 and 2 contained 6 mice per group; there were 5 mice per group in Experiment 3.

[b] RIL-2 was injected intraperitoneally approximately every 8 hr from days 3 through 8 after tumor injection; mice received 7,500, 6,000, and 25,000 units per injection in Experiments 1, 2, and 3, respectively.

[c] LAK cells received 3,000 rad in a γ irradiator before i.v. injection on days 3 and 6 after tumor injection; 1×10^8 LAK cells were given each time.

[d] Statistical significance of differences: Experiment 1 A vs · B, NS; C, NS; D, $p < 0.005$; E, NS. B vs.: C, NS; D, $p < 0.005$; E, NS. C vs.: D, $p < 0.005$; E, NS. D vs.: E, < 0.005. Experiment 2. A vs.: D, $p < 0.005$; E, $p < 0.005$. D vs.: E, $p < 0.005$. Experiment 3. A vs.: B, NS; D, $p < 0.01$; E, NS. B vs.: D, $p < 0.01$; E, NS. D vs.: E, $p < 0.01$.

From Mule, J. J. et al., *J. Immunol.*, 135, 646, 1985. With permission.

Table 13
TISSUE-SPECIFIC LYMPHOID PROLIFERATION IN MICE RECEIVING LAK CELLS AND IL-2

	CPM ± SEM[a] (PI)[b]			
Organ	HBSS[c]	IL-2[c]	LAK[d] + HBSS	LAK + IL-2
Lung	429 ± 24 (−)	1300 ± 469 (3.0)	1080 ± 60 (2.5)	3824 ± 916 (8.9)
Liver	2920 ± 702 (−)	5410 ± 1991 (1.9)	3833 ± 1511 (1.3)	17388 ± 6510 (6.0)
Kidney	830 ± 135 (−)	1592 ± 321 (1.9)	1267 ± 476 (1.5)	8663 ± 7017 (10.4)
Spleen	1570 ± 368 (−)	4438 ± 2220 (2.8)	4349 ± 4761 (2.8)	14656 ± 2829 (9.3)

[a] Mean counts per minute ± standard error of organs of 3 mice per treatment group harvested on day 7 after starting IL-2 treatment.

[b] Proliferation index (PI) equals CPM of organs from experimentally treated mice divided by mean CPM of organs from HBSS treated mice.

[c] IL-2 6000 units (or HBSS) in 0.5 mℓ i.p. 3 times a day from day 0 through 7.

[d] LAK 10^8 cells in HBSS 1 mℓ i.v. on day 0.

From Ettinghausen, S. E. et al., *J. Immunol.*, 135, 3623, 1985. With permission.

kidneys, and spleen on day 7 from a representative experiment are presented in Table 13. In each organ, RIL-2 alone induced increased incorporation of ^{125}IUdR. The transfer of LAK cells alone produced a transient, though small increase in ^{125}IUdR incorporation in lungs, liver, and kidneys with a greater increase in spleen. Administration of LAK cells plus RIL-2 led to a greater ^{125}IUdR uptake in lungs, liver, spleen, and kidneys than did treatment with either alone. The increased ^{125}IUdR incorporation into tissues in mice receiving LAK cells plus RIL-2 compared to that of RIL-2 alone or cells alone was dependent on in vitro activation of LAK cell activity by RIL-2 prior to cell

Table 14
IN VITRO CYTOTOXICITY OF ADOPTIVELY TRANSFERRED LAK CELLS RECOVERED FROM RECIPIENT LUNGS[a]

Treatment of mice	Number of lymphocytes recovered per mouse ($\times 10^{-6}$)	Percent lysis[c] (effector to target ratio = 100:1/20:1)	Lytic units[d] per 10^6 cells	Lytic units per lungs
HBSS[b]	0.6	5.4/7.8	<1	<1
IL-2[b]	0.7	22.5/17.7	<1	<1
LAK + HBSS	1.6	78.7/31.2	8.8	14.4
LAK + IL-2	52.8	86.1/27.4	8.8	463.4

[a]   Whole body irradiated (500 rad) mice received 10^8 LAK cells intravenously on day 0 or no cells.
[b]   IL-2 200,000 units (or HBSS) intraperitoneally 3 times a day from day 0 through 3.
[c]   Lymphocytes isolated from lungs of treated mice were used as effectors in an 18 hr ^{51}Cr release assay against a fresh murine sarcoma target. Standard in vitro generated LAK cells were employed as a positive control in the assay and produced 185 lytic units per 10^6 cells.
[d]   One lytic unit defined as number of effectors to produce 50% lysis of 3×10^3 tumor target cells.

From Ettinghausen, S. E. et al., *J. Immunol.*, 135, 3623, 1985. With permission.

injection.[50] The i.v. transfer of fresh splenocytes or splenocytes cultured in vitro for 3 days in medium without RIL-2 resulted in markedly less ^{125}IUdR incorporation that did injection of LAK cells. In all experiments, RIL-2 administration alone caused an increase in proliferation in tissues, though generally less than that seen when LAK cells plus RIL-2 were injected. In an attempt to differentiate proliferation of endogenous lymphoid cells from that of injected LAK cells, mice were given 500 rad total body irradiation immediately prior to cell transfer and/or RIL-2 administration. We found that in preirradiated mice, IL-2 dependent proliferation of exogenous LAK cells was largely preserved, but the proliferation attributed to high dose RIL-2 alone was largely eliminated.[50] Further, the irradiation of LAK cells with 3000 rad prior to cell transfer eliminated the tissue proliferation seen in conjunction with RIL-2. These results argued that the increased proliferation seen in the tissues of mice receiving LAK cells plus RIL-2 was due to division of the injected LAK cells, themselves.

The simplest hypothesis to explain these observations involves the traffic of injected LAK cells to the tumor site followed by the expansion of these lytic cells locally under the influence of exogenously administered RIL-2. Further supporting this hypothesis are our experiments performed using the adoptive transfer of Thy-1.2 congenic LAK cells into mice bearing the Thy-1.1 allele[50] and the histologic studies which have sequentially analyzed the cellular events at the site of tumor destruction when high doses of RIL-2 are administered. The infiltration of activated lymphocytes into the tumor stroma with subsequent tumor destruction argues for a direct role of these activated lymphocytes in tumor cell killing. Alternatively, these activated lymphocytes may be producing other lymphokines which either have antitumor effects directly or which provide chemotactic factors that allow for an influx of other cells with lytic capability.

Since it was not clear whether LAK cells themselves or a nonlytic T-cell population derived from the bulk, transferred lymphocytes were proliferating in vivo in response to RIL-2, we assayed the in vivo cytotoxicity of LAK cells isolated from the lungs of treated mice. Whole body irradiated (500 rad) mice received 1×10^8 LAK cells i.v. (or no cells) on day 0. RIL-2 200,000 units (or HBSS) was administered until day 3 at which time the animals were sacrificed the lymphoid cells recovered from the lungs.[50] An 18 hr ^{51}Cr-release assay was performed using the isolated lymphocytes as effectors.

As shown in Table 14, the transfer of LAK cells to mice followed by repeated injec-

Table 15
SUMMARY OF FINDINGS

1. LAK cells show broad lytic specificity in vitro to a variety of fresh tumor cells but do not lyse fresh normal cells.
2. Successful regression of established pulmonary and hepatic metastases can be achieved by the adoptive transfer of LAK cells plus RIL-2.
3. The adoptive transfer of fresh or unstimulated splenocytes have no antimetastatic effect; a 2 to 3 day incubation of splenocytes in RIL-2 is required.
4. The efficacy of therapy is directly related to the dose of LAK cells and the amount of RIL-2 administered.
5. Allogeneic LAK cells are effective cells in adoptive immunotherapy.
6. Metastases from 3 different sarcomas, 2 melanomas, and a colon adenocarcinoma have been successfully treated, some of which have little, or no immunogenicity.
7. Irradiated LAK cells have a reduced antimetastatic capacity.
8. The combined therapy of LAK cells plus RIL-2 is highly effective in mice immunosuppressed by sublethal total body irradiation and in T-cell depleted mice.
9. Adoptively transferred LAK cells divide in vivo when RIL-2 is administered concomitantly.
10. Adoptively transferred LAK cells can be isolated from recipient lungs during regression of established pulmonary metastases.
11. High doses of RIL-2 alone can mediate therapeutic effects though the magnitude of reduction in metastases is greater when LAK cells are also administered.
12. Systemic administration of high doses of RIL-2 generates LAK cells in vivo that can be isolated from the lung, liver, and spleen of treated mice.
13. Larger, established 10-day pulmonary metastases are more susceptible to the effects of RIL-2 than are smaller, 3-day pulmonary metastases.
14. The antitumor effects of the systemic administration of RIL-2 are eliminated if mice receive prior treatment with 500 rads total body irradiation.

tions of IL-2 lead to a substantial increase in the number of recovered lymphocytes when compared to mice receiving LAK cells and HBSS, RIL-2 alone or HBSS alone. Highly lytic lymphoid cells were obtained from the lungs of mice receiving LAK cells with or without RIL-2 [8.8 lytic units (L.U.) per 10^6 cells compared to mice treated with HBSS or RIL-2 alone (<1 L.U.)]. However, the higher recovery of lymphocytes from the LAK cell and RIL-2 treated animals yielded a significantly greater number of L.U. per mouse when compared with the LAK cell and HBSS treated group (463.4 and 14.4 L.U., respectively). Thus, the expanding cells seen in mice receiving LAK cells and RIL-2 have the capability to lyse both tumor target cells and are consistent with our functional definition of LAK cells. Further, these lytic cells can also be recovered in large numbers from the lungs of mice during the regression of established pulmonary metastases.[47]

VI. CONCLUSIONS

The use of specifically immune cells in adoptive immunotherapy has received very little attention in humans, largely because of the difficulty associated with generating large numbers of specifically reactive cells for adoptive transfer. The experimental evidence for the existence of lymphocyte-mediated reactions in humans to unique or shared tumor associated antigens capable of causing tumor destruction in vivo or in vitro is inconclusive. This lack of specific lymphocyte reactivity may be related, in part, to the poor (or absent) immunogenicity of human tumors and the difficulty in identifying and isolating those lymphocytes, of low incidence, with tumor specificity.

In this review we have described our approach to developing an adoptive immunotherapy that may be applicable to the treatment of human cancer. Extensive studies of the adoptive immunotherapy of established lung and liver metastases with the combination of LAK cells plus RIL-2 and of the systemic administration of high-dose RIL-2 alone have been conducted.[38-43,47,48] A summary of the findings of our therapy experiments, and of the possible mechanism operational in vivo, is presented in Table 15.

The adoptive transfer of LAK cells now appears to be an effective alternative approach to the use of specifically immune cells in the therapy of established metastases of a variety of cancers, regardless of the immunogenicity of the tumor in vivo. By using IL-2, human LAK cells with in vitro properties identical to those of murine LAK cells can readily be generated in vitro. Further, the availability of large amounts of recombinant IL-2 with known biologic activity, has now made it feasible to evaluate this immunotherapeutic approach in humans. Clinical trials are currently underway to test the efficacy of treatment with LAK cells plus RIL-2 in humans with established cancer.

REFERENCES

1. Rosenberg, S. A. and Terry, W., Passive immunotherapy of cancer in animals and man, *Adv. Cancer Res.*, 25, 323, 1977.
2. Berendt, M. J. and North, R. J., T-cell mediated suppression of anti-tumor immunity. An explanation for progressive growth of an immunogenic tumor, *J. Exp. Med.*, 151, 69, 1980.
3. Borberg, H., Oettgen, H. F., Choudry, K., and Beattie, E. J., Inhibition of established transplants of chemically induced sarcomas in syngeneic mice by lymphocytes from immunized donors, *Int. J. Cancer*, 10, 539, 1972.
4. Cheever, M. A., Kempf, R. A., and Fefer, A., Tumor neutralization, immunotherapy, and chemoimmunotherapy of a friend leukemia with cells secondarily sensitized *in vitro*, *J. Immunol.*, 119, 714, 1977.
5. Fernandez-Cruz, E., Halliburton, B., and Feldman, J. D., *In vivo* elimination by specific effector cells of an established syngeneic rat Moloney virus-induced sarcoma, *J. Immunol.*, 123, 1772, 1979.
6. Kedar, E. and Weiss, D. W., The *in vitro* generation of effector lymphocytes and their employment in tumor immunotherapy, *Adv. Cancer Res.*, 38, 171, 1983.
7. Shu, S., Fonseca, L. S., Kato, H., and Zbar, B., Mechanisms of immunological eradication of syngeneic guinea pig tumor: participation of a component(s) of recipient origin in the expression of systemic adoptive immunity, *Cancer Res.*, 43, 2637, 1983.
8. Smith, H. G., Harmel, R. P., Hanna, M. G., Zwilling, B. S., Zbar, B., and Rapp, H. J., Regression of established intradermal tumors and lymph node metastases in guinea pigs after systemic transfer of immune lymphoid cells, *J. Natl. Cancer Inst.*, 58, 1315, 1977.
9. Delorme, E. J., Treatment of primary fibrosarcoma in the rat with immune lymphocytes, *Lancet*, 7, 117, 1984.
10. Fefer, A., Einstein, A. B., Jr., Cheever, M. A., and Berenson, J. R., Models for syngeneic adoptive chemoimmunotherapy of murine leukemias, *Ann. N.Y. Acad. Sci.*, 277, 492, 1976.
11. Berendt, M. J., and North, R. J., T cell-mediated suppression of antitumor immunity. An explanation for progressive growth of an immunogenic tumor, *J. Exp. Med.*, 151, 69, 1980.
12. Eberlein, T. J., Rosenstein, M., and Rosenberg, S. A., Regression of a disseminated syngeneic solid tumor by systemic transfer of lymphoid cells expanded in IL-2, *J. Exp. Med.*, 156, 385, 1982.
13. Rosenstein, M., Eberlein, T. J., and Rosenberg, S. A., Adoptive immunotherapy of established syngeneic solid tumors: role of T lymphoid subpopulations, *J. Immunol.*, 132, 2117, 1984.
14. North, R. J., Dye, E. S., and Mills, C. D., T cell-mediated negative regulation of concomitant antitumor immunity as an obstacle to adoptive immunotherapy of established tumors, in *The Potential Role of T Cell Populations in Cancer Therapy*, Fefer, A. and Goldstein, A. L., Eds., Raven Press, New York, 1981, 65.
15. Hellström, K. E., Hellström, I., Kant, J. A., and Tamerius, J., Regression and inhibition of sarcoma growth by interference with a radiosensitive T-cell population, *J. Exp. Med.*, 148, 799, 1978.
16. Hellström, K. E. and Hellström, I., Cell-mediated suppression of tumor immunity has a nonspecific component. I. Evidence from transplantation tests, *Int. J. Cancer*, 27, 481, 1981.
17. Grimm, E. A., Vose, B. M., Chu, E. W., Wilson, D. J., Lotze, M. T., Rayner, A. A., and Rosenberg, S. A., The human mixed lymphocyte-tumor interaction test. I. Positive autologous lymphocyte proliferative responses can be stimulated by tumor cells as well as by cells from normal tissues, *Cancer Immunol. Immunother.*, 17, 83, 1984.
18. Rosenberg, S. A., Rosenstein, M., Grimm, E., Lotze, M. T., and Mazumder, A., The use of lymphoid cells expanded in IL-2 for the adoptive immunotherapy of murine and human tumors, in *Thymic Hormones and Lymphokines*, Goldstein, A. L., Ed., Plenum Press, New York, 1984, 191.

19. Rosenberg, S. A., Adoptive immunotherapy of cancer: accomplishments and prospects, *Cancer Treat. Rep.*, 68, 233, 1984.

20. Rosenberg, S. A., Shu, S., and Mulé, J. J., Approaches to the adoptive immunotherapy of cancer, in *Manipulation of Host Defense Mechanisms,* Aoki, T., Tsubura, E., and Urushizaki, I., Eds., Excerpta Med., p70, 1984.

21. Yron, I., Wood, T. A., Spiess, P., and Rosenberg, S. A., *In vitro* growth of murine T-cells. V. The isolation and growth of lymphoid cells infiltrating syngeneic solid tumors, *J. Immunol.*, 125, 238, 1980.

22. Lotze, M. T., Grimm, E., Mazumder, A., Strausser, J. L., and Rosenberg, S. A., *In vitro* growth of cytotoxic human lymphocytes. IV. Lysis of fresh and cultured autologous tumor by lymphocytes cultured in T cell growth factor (TCGF), *Cancer Res.*, 41, 4420, 1981.

23. Grimm, E. A., Robb, R. J., Roth, J. A., Neckers, L. M., Lachman, L. B., Wilson, D. J., and Rosenberg, S. A., Lymphokine-activated killer cell (LAK) phenomenon. III. Evidence that IL-2 alone is sufficient for direct activation of PBL into LAK, *J. Exp. Med.*, 158, 1356, 1983.

24. Rosenberg, S. A., Grimm, E. A., McGrogan, M., Doyle, M., Kawasaki, E., Koths, K., and Mark, D. F., Biological activity of recombinant human interleukin-2 produced in E. Coli, *Science*, 223, 1412, 1984.

25. Rosenstein, M., Yron, I., Kaufmann, Y., and Rosenberg, S. A., Lymphokine activated killer cells: lysis of fresh syngeneic NK-resistant murine tumor cells by lymphocytes cultured in interleukin-2, *Cancer Res.*, 44, 1946, 1984.

26. Grimm, E. A., Mazumder, A., Zhang, H. Z., and Rosenberg, S. A., The lymphokine activated killer cell phenomenon: lysis of NK resistant fresh solid tumor cells by IL-2 activated autologous human peripheral blood lymphocytes, *J. Exp. Med.*, 155, 1823, 1982.

27. Grimm,. E. A., Ramsey, K. M., Mazumder, A., Wilson, D. J., Djen, J. Y., and Rosenberg, S. A., Lymphokine-activated killer cell phenomenon. II. The precursor phenotype is serologically distinct from peripheral T lymphocytes, memory CTL, and NK cells, *J. Exp. Med.*, 157, 884, 1983.

28. Grimm, E. A., and Rosenberg, S. A., The human lymphokine-activated killer cell phenomenon, in *Lymphokines,* Vol. 9, Academic Press, Orlando, Fla., 1984, p. 279.

29. Mazumder, A. and Rosenberg, S. A., Lysis of fresh human solid tumors by activated autologous lymphocytes: potential applications to tumor immunotherapy, in *Rational Basis for Chemotherapy,* Alan R. Liss, New York, 1983, p 359.

30. Rosenberg, S. A., Guest editorial: lymphokine-activated killer cells: a new approach to the immunotherapy of cancer, *J. Natl. Cancer Inst.*, 75, 595, 1985.

31. Mazumder, A. M., Grimm, E. A., Zhang, H. Z., and Rosenberg, S. A., Lysis of fresh human solid tumors by autologous lymphocytes activated *in vitro* with lectins., *Cancer Res.*, 42, 913, 1982.

32. Zarling, J. M., Robins, H. I., Raich, P. C., Bach, F. H., and Bach, M. L., Generation of cytotoxic T lymphocytes to human leukemia cells by sensitization to pooled allogeneic normal cells, *Nature (London)*, 274, 269, 1978.

33. Strausser, J. L., Mazumder, A., Grimm, E. A., Lotze, M. T., and Rosenberg, S. A., Lysis of human solid tumors by autologous cells sensitized *in vitro* to alloantigens, *J. Immunol.*, 127, 266, 1981.

34. Mazumder, A., Grimm, E. A., and Rosenberg, S. A., The lysis of fresh human solid tumors by autologous lymphocytes activated *in vitro* by allosensitization, *Cancer Immunol. Immunother.*, 15, 1, 1983.

35. Zielski, J. V. and Golub, S. H., Fetal calf serum-induced blastogenic and cytotoxic response of human lymphocytes, *Cancer Res.*, 36, 3842, 1976.

36. Donohue, J. H. and Rosenberg, S. A., The fate of interleukin-2 following *in vivo* administration, *J. Immunol.*, 130, 2203, 1983.

37. Taniguchi, T., Matsui, H., Fajita, T., Takaoki, C., Kashina, N., Yoshimoto, R., and Hamuro, J., Structure and expression of a cloned cDNA for human interleukin-2, *Nature (London)*, 302, 305, 1983.

38. Mulé, J. J., Shu, S., Schwarz, S. L., and Rosenberg, S. A., Adoptive immunotherapy of established pulmonary metastases with LAK cells and recombinant interleukin-2, *Science*, 225, 1487, 1984.

39. Mulé, J. J., Shu, S., and Rosenberg, S. A., The anti-tumor efficacy of lymphokine-activated killer cells and recombinant interleukin-2 *in vivo, J. Immunol.*, 135, 646, 1985.

40. Rosenberg, S. A., and Mulé, J. J., Immunotherapy of cancer with lymphokine-activated killer cells and recombinant interleukin-2, *Surgery,* 98, 437, 1985.

41. Lafreniere, R. and Rosenberg, S. A., Successful immunotherapy of experimental hepatic metastases with lymphokine-activated killer cells and recombinant interleukin-2, *Cancer Res.*, 45, 3735, 1985.

42. Lafreniere, R., and Rosenberg, S. A., Adoptive immunotherapy of murine hepatic metastases with lymphokine activated killer (LAK) cells and recombinant interleukin-2 (RIL-2) can mediate the regression of both immunogenic and nonimmunogenic sarcomas and an adenocarcinoma, *J. Immunol.*, 135, 4243, 1985.

43. Mulé, J. J., Ettinghausen, S. E., Spiess, P. J., Shu, S., and Rosenberg, S. A., The antitumor efficacy of lymphokine-activated killer cells and recombinant IL-2 *in vivo:* an analysis of survival benefit and mechanisms of tumor escape in mice undergoing immunotherapy, *Cancer Res.,* 46, 676, 1985.

44. Mazumder, A. and Rosenberg, S. A., Successful immunotherapy of natural killer-resistant established pulmonary melanoma metastases by the intravenous adoptive transfer of syngeneic lymphocytes activated *in vitro* by interleukin-2, *J. Exp. Med.,* 159, 495, 1984.

45. Greenberg, P. D., Cheever, M. A., and Fefer, A., H-2 restriction of adoptive immunotherapy of advanced tumors, *J. Immunol.,* 126, 2100, 1981.

46. Chang, A. E., Hyatt, C. L., and Rosenberg, S. A., Systemic administration of recombinant IL-2 in mice, *J. Biol. Resp. Modif.,* 3, 561, 1984.

47. Mulé, J. J., Yang, J., Shu, S., and Rosenberg, S. A., The anti-tumor efficacy of lymphokine-activated killer cells and recombinant interleukin-2 *in vivo:* direct correlation between reduction of established metastases and *in vitro* cytolytic activity of lymphokine-activated killer cells, *J. Immunol.,* 136, 3899, 1986.

48. Rosenberg, S. A., Mulé, J. J., Spiess, P. J., Reichert, C. M., and Schwarz, S. L., Regression of established pulmonary metastases and subcutaneous tumor mediated by the systemic administration of high-dose recombinant interleukin-2, *J. Exp. Med.,* 161, 1169, 1985.

49. Ettinghausen, S. E., Lipford, E. H., III, Mulé, J. J., and Rosenberg, S. A., Systemic administration of recombinant interleukin 2 stimulates *in vivo* lymphoid cell proliferation in tissues, *J. Immunol.,* 135, 1488, 1985.

50. Ettinghausen, S. E., Lipford, E. H., III, Mulé, J. J., and Rosenberg, S. A., Recombinant interleukin 2 stimulates *in vivo* proliferation of adoptively transferred lymphokine activated killer (LAK) cells, *J. Immunol.,* 135, 3623, 1986.

Chapter 12

BASIC AND APPLIED PRINCIPLES OF ACTIVE SPECIFIC IMMUNO-THERAPY IN THE TREATMENT OF METASTATIC SOLID TUMORS

M. G. Hanna, Jr. and H. C. Hoover, Jr.

TABLE OF CONTENTS

I. INTRODUCTION

Immunotherapy encompasses the relationship of the immune system to the control of neoplastic growth. The central hypothesis underlying specific immunotherapy is that tumor cells express immunogenic determinants not associated with normal adult tissues. For the immune system to be operative and for immunotherapy to be effective, tumor cells must be immunogenic in the autochthonous host. The existence of tumor-associated antigen(s) that provoke tumor rejection by humoral and/or cell-mediated responses in the host is a distinct characteristic of experimental chemically or virally induced tumors.[1-3] The tumor-associated antigens of experimental tumors have generally been detected by classic transplantation techniques. However, detection of tumor-associated antigen(s) of spontaneous tumors has been more difficult. The failure to detect these antigen(s) in many experimental spontaneous tumor systems[4,5] has resulted in speculations that immune systems can fail to recognize neoplastic cells or that neoplastic growth can occur despite the presence of host response. Why the host system is not effective or even operative under certain conditions is a major question in tumor immunology.[6]

The development of antitumor immunity is an intricate immunological process that is subject to a series of specific and nonspecific feedback mechanisms involving the generation of suppressor T-cells and macrophages. Tumor cells, depending on the method of presentation, can be both immunogenic and immunosuppressive.[7] Peripheral-blood mononuclear cells harvested from about one third of the patients with colorectal carcinoma either lyse tumor cells,[8,9] or proliferate when cultured with autologous tumor cells.[10] The evidence that sets of lymphocytes and macrophages suppress the response to tumor-associated antigens of experimental neoplasms[11-14] in test animals suggests that suppressor cells may exist that have a similar function in human patients. Other studies have demonstrated that when suppressor cells are depleted from human peripheral blood mononuclear cells, effector cells can lyse autologous osteosarcoma cells;[15] therefore, although tumor-associated antigens may be immunogenic for autochthonous hosts, suppressor cells may inhibit the response to tumor-associated antigens and, in the process, make the tumor appear to be nonimmunogenic. Clearly, there is much still to be learned about tumor-associated antigens and the complexities of the host immune response.

Tumor immunology has been in a decade-long struggle during which implementation of biological therapy as an adjunct to standard cancer treatment has been the unrealized goal. Immunotherapy, a category of biological therapy, gained popularity as a treatment in the 1960s because of data from experimental tumor models that indicated that both specific stimulation of the immune system with antigen-bearing tumor cells and nonspecific stimulation with bacteria, viruses, and other adjuvant-type compounds could enhance the immune response in animals and prevent recurrence or delay growth of experimentally transplanted tumors. Thus, the method of presentation and stimulation of the afferent and efferent immune response was shown to require the presumptive tumor-associated antigens as well as immunomodulators. Since immunotherapy was most effective against small tumor burdens, investigators began to study immunotherapy as a possible treatment for minimal residual disease. These studies were based on the premise that treatment of animals with minimal residual disease would be analogous to postsurgical treatment of cancer in humans. Since further improvements in surgical techniques were unlikely to produce vastly improved cure rates because anatomically defined limits have already been reached for the excision of most tumors and since adjuvant chemotherapy and radiation therapy played relatively minor roles in the adjunct treatment of cancer because the tumors developed resistance to the therapy or because toxicity limits dosage,[16,17] new strategies of immunotherapy for treatment of metastatic solid tumors were desperately needed. However, the analogies from the animal system were frequently stretched beyond the limits of sound logic. Artificially induced foci of tumor cells were not representative of the well-vascularized metastasis of the cancer patient. Given the variability of clinical presentation, it is not surprising that randomized trials of immunotherapy did not succeed in reducing the incidence of recurrent cancer. Although the overall clinical experience with immunotherapy has not resulted in the development of definitive treatments, one must recognize that not all immunotherapy studies have been negative.[18] Some randomized controlled studies report positive results which indicate the need for adequately designed protocols based on a fundamental understanding of the biology of cancer. In the following discussions, we concentrate on certain fundamentals of the biology of cancer and tumor immunology which should guide us in the development of future approaches to multimodal treatment of metastatic solid cancer.

II. EXPERIMENTAL STUDIES OF ACTIVE SPECIFIC IMMUNOTHERAPY IN THE GUINEA PIG TUMOR MODEL

A. Development and Modification of the Guinea Pig Tumor Model

A major contribution to understanding the principles of active specific immunotherapy has been the development and biological characterization of an adequate experimental model that fulfills the requirements for studying effective immunotherapy of established tumors.

Our early studies demonstrated that when strain-2 guinea pigs bearing a transplanted syngeneic line-10 (L10) hepatocarcinoma were given intratumoral injections of viable Bacillus Calmette Guérin (BCG), the primary tumor regressed and regional metastases were eliminated.[19,21] In the course of this reaction, systemic tumor immunity developed. Further studies showed that this immunity was effective in eradicating both regional and systemic malignancies.[22,23]

However, this intratumor model of immunotherapy was limited by the fact that most human tumors are not accessible to direct injection. Consequently, we modified the guinea pig hepatocarcinoma model to make it more relevant to the clinical situation. A tumor cell vaccine consisting of L10 tumor cells and BCG was developed and shown to successfully stimulate systemic tumor immunity in strain-2 guinea pigs. A series of studies[24-39] demonstrated that BCG, admixed with tumor cells, could induce a degree of systemic tumor immunity that would eliminate a small, disseminated tumor burden (Figures 1 and 2) when the vaccine was carefully controlled for such variables as the number of viable, but nontumorigenic tumors cells (10^7 optimal), the ratio of viable BCG organisms to tumor cells (1:1); and the vaccine regimen (3 vaccines, 1 week apart) was carefully administered (Table 1). Most prior clinical trials of tumor vaccines used either nonviable (metabolically inactive) autologous tumor cells or allogeneic tumor cells; both were found to be totally ineffective in the guinea pig.

The percentage of viable tumor cells in the vaccine was strongly correlated with the efficacy of the vaccine. Vaccines with low tumor cell viability (less than 50%) were less effective than vaccines with high tumor cell viability (greater than 70%). The latter was best achieved with proper tumor-cell dissociation procedures and optimal cryopreservation techniques.[32] Another important factor in vaccine efficacy was dose of adjuvant (Figure 3). Variation in dose of either *Corynebacterium parvum* or BCG, with constant tumor cell dose (10^7), had a marked influence on percentage survival of vaccinated guinea pigs injected with L10 cells. In general, the low adjuvant mixture was ineffective and more adjuvant (>70 μg/ *C. parvum* or $>10^7$ BCG) was not proportionately beneficial.

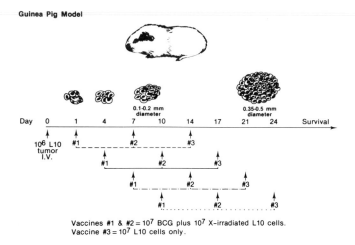

Vaccines #1 & #2 = 10^7 BCG plus 10^7 X-irradiated L10 cells.
Vaccine #3 = 10^7 L10 cells only.

FIGURE 1.   Experimental studies of active specific immunotherapy in the guinea pig tumor model system: schema.

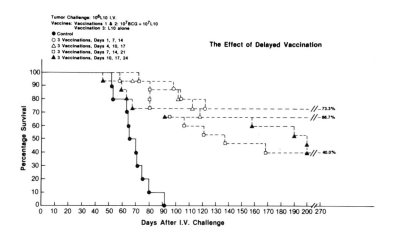

FIGURE 2.   Experimental studies of active specific immunotherapy in the guinea pig tumor model system: percentage survival as a function of time after challenge.

B. Studies on the Effect of Anatomic Characteristics of Tumor Foci on Host-Tumor Interaction

Using the L10 hepatocarcinoma as a model tumor system, we investigated some mechanisms by which tumors evade host defense systems. These studies suggested that the anatomic characteristics of the developing tumor foci restrict various aspects of the host-tumor interaction. These restrictions may protect tumors not only from immunotherapy but from other forms of treatment as well.

Research into mechanisms by which tumors evade the immune system has focused primarily on the poor immunogenicity of spontaneous tumors or the immune incompetence of the host. Less attention has been given to the possibility that the anatomic characteristics of tumor foci might restrict host-tumor interactions, thus protecting tumors not only from immunotherapy, but from other forms of treatment as well.[40,41] Recent studies have shown that blood-borne antitumor antibodies do not penetrate uniformly into all growing areas of solid tumors, but are restricted to those areas of the tumors that are highly vascularized, or hemorrhagic.[42,43] In some cases, the inabil-

Table 1
VACCINES FOR ACTIVE SPECIFIC IMMUNOTHERAPY

Adjuvant
    A. BCG (Phipps, Tice, Connaught): lyophilized, frozen (dose-dependence $> 10^6 = 10^7 - 10^8$)
    B. *C. parvum* (Wellcome Labs) (dose-dependence $>7 \mu g = 70 \mu g < 700 \mu g$)

Tumor Cells
    A. Enzymatic dissociation
        1. Collagenase type I (1.5 − 2.0 units/mℓ HBSS[a])
        2. DNase (450 K.U./mℓ HBSS)
        3. 37°C with stirring
    B. Cryopreservation
        1. Controlled-rate freezing (−1°C/min) (7.5% DMSO[b], 5% FBS[c], HBSS)
        2. Viability ≥ 80%
    C. X-irradiation
        1. Rendered nontumorigenic at 12,000 to 20,000 R

Components and Administration[d]
    A. Ratio of adjuvant to tumor cells — 10:1-1:1 (optimum)
    B. 10^7 tumor cells (optimum)
    C. 2 to 3 intradermal vaccinations at weekly intervals (3rd vaccination contains tumor cells only)

[a]   HBSS, Hank's balanced salt solution.
[b]   DMSO, dimethyl sulfoxide.
[c]   FBS, fetal bovine.
[d]   Inhibition of chemoprophylaxis of BCG infection optional.

ity of antibody to penetrate all areas of the tumor has been associated with the ability of the tumor to survive a potentially lethal attack.[44] Other blood-borne substances, such as chemotherapeutic agents, also encounter similar barriers, thus limiting their access to all portions of the tumors.[45,46] Such vascular barriers may provide an environment in which some tumor cells survive blood-borne chemotherapeutic and biologic agents. Studies have shown that the penetration of drugs into avascular tumor spheroids of 0.25 mm diameter is poor,[45] and that solid tumors as small as 1 mm in diameter frequently contain areas that are poorly vascularized.[46] This latter characteristic of microscopic metastatic foci could not only limit effectiveness of immune effector components and cytotoxic drugs, but in the case of the latter, could increase the chance of drug-resistant cell development because of the exposure of some cells to subtherapeutic amounts of the drug. In addition, solid tumor nodules may serve as "pharmacologic sanctuaries", allowing even drug-sensitive tumor cells to continue to grow. Either or both of these factors may result in continued tumor growth and lead to the conclusion that the tumor is drug resistant.

Our morphologic studies in guinea pigs vaccinated with L10 hepatocarcinoma cells revealed that host cell-mediated hypersensitivity reactions occurred at the sites of pulmonary metastasis in the immunized guinea pigs.[47] These nodules were infiltrated by a predominantly mononuclear cell population made up of lymphocytes and the cells of the macrophage-histiocyte series (Figure 4). This infiltration disrupted the typical compact architecture of the tumor foci (Figure 5). Karyorexis and cytolysis were detected only after the inflammatory disruption of the established metastatic tumor nodules had occurred, suggesting that the tumor cells were killed by the same effector cells that had

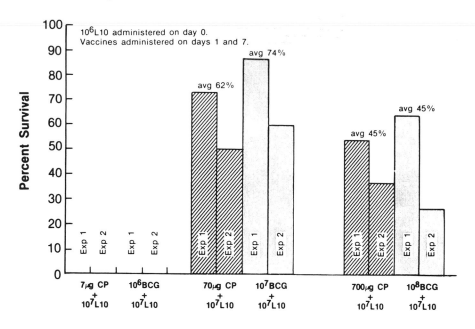

FIGURE 3.   Efficacy of various doses of *Corynebacterium parvum* and BCG as adjuvants in L10 tumor cell vaccines.

earlier infiltrated and disrupted the nodules. Presumably, some of the infiltrating lymphocytes were sensitized to TAA. These effector cells have been shown to be not only tumoricidal but also to produce lymphokines and cytokines in the presence of specific antigens.[48] These factors are chemotactic for mononuclear cells and initiate inflammatory tissue reactions which may have contributed to the disruption of the nodules.[48] Eventually these tumor foci were transformed into chronic inflammatory lesions with histiocytosis and ischemic necrosis. Thus, the observed tumor killing apparently was correlated with the development of a cell-mediated immune response and anatomic disruption of the micrometastatic nodules.

The nature of the anatomic alterations in metastatic nodules that accompany active specific immunotherapy was explored further by use of an anti-L10 monoclonal antibody (D3) as a probe to assess vascular permeability within tumors.[49-51] The tumor-specific monoclonal antibody was injected intravenously into either untreated or vaccinated tumor-bearing guinea pigs at a time determined histologically to be peak of the cell-mediated hypersensitivity reaction in the metastatic nodules. The D3 monoclonal antibody was chosen because of its ability to bind to a TAA and to remain localized at the site of extravasation for extended periods of time. After injection of the D3 antibody, an immunoperoxidase-staining technique was used to localize the monoclonal antibody within metastases. Morphometric analysis of antibody distribution showed that significantly more antibody accumulated in tumors of vaccinated guinea pigs than in comparable tumors of untreated guinea pigs. Furthermore, the average distance between a given tumor cell and a histologically identifiable blood vessel in metastases of untreated guinea pigs was significantly greater than the average distance between a given tumor cell and an identifiable blood vessel in metastases of vaccinated guinea pigs (Table 2).

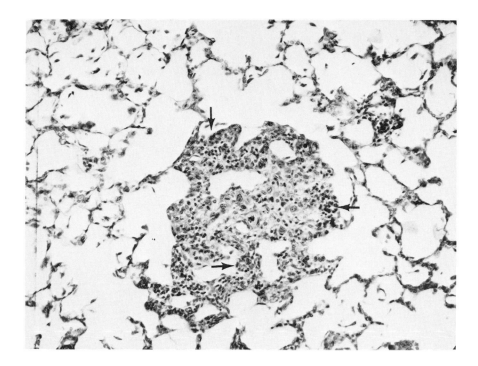

FIGURE 4. Metastatic L10 tumor nodule in the lung of a guinea pig 7 days after the first vaccination (14 days after tumor challenge). The nodule is being infiltrated by mononuclear cells. Arrows indicate lymphocyte and macrophage concentrations (hematoxylin and eosin; × 185).

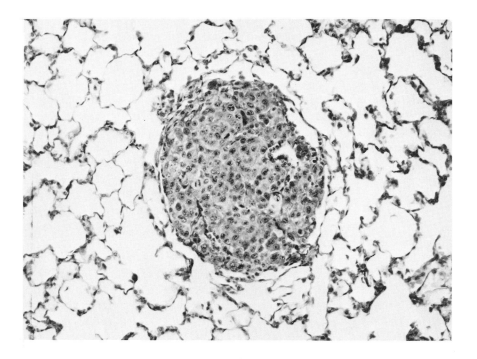

FIGURE 5. Metastatic nodule in the lung of a control guinea pig 21 days after i.v. injection of L10 cells. The nodule (diameter, 0.35 mm) has numerous mitotic figures and is highly vascularized. There is no evidence of host cell-mediated inflammation (hematoxylin and eosin; × 185).

Table 2

VASCULAR PATTERNS AND PERMEABILITY IN PULMONARY MATASTASES OF THE LINE 10 HEPATOCARCINOMA AFTER IMMUNOTHERAPY AND CHEMOTHERAPY

Tumor source[a]	Tumors positive[b] for D3 antibody	Average distance[c] between tumor cells and blood vessels (μm)
Untreated controls	8 ± 12^d	58 ± 19
Vaccinated guinea pig	63 ± 16^d	32 ± 14^e
Drug-treated guinea pig	31 ± 23^d	ND[f]

[a]   Guinea pigs bearing pulmonary line 10 tumors received no further treatment (untreated controls), received immunotherapy on days 10, 17, and 24 (vaccinated), or received cyclophosphamide on day 31 (drug-treated).

[b]   D3 antibody was injected intravenously on day 31 into untreated and vaccinated guinea pigs and on day 38 in drug-treated guinea pigs. Lungs were removed 24 hr later, and distribution of D3 antibody in the pulmonary metastases was analyzed.

[c]   Distances were measured on photographic enlargements of tumors.

[d]   All three values are significantly different from each other ($p < 0.01$; Duncan's multiple range test).

[e]   Significantly different from untreated controls ($p = 0.008$; student's t-test). Values are the means $\pm$ SD for a total of 10 untreated tumors, 8 vaccine-treated tumors, and 10 drug-treated tumors.

[f]   ND, not done.

C. Studies on Combination Therapies

These findings suggested that a treatment strategy that combined active specific immunotherapy with the i.v. delivery of cytotoxic substances, such as chemotherapeutic agents, monoclonal antibodies, and immunoconjugates, might be more effective than any single approach.

To test this hypothesis, we challenged strain-2 guinea pigs intravenously with 10^6 L10 cells (100 times the minimum lethal dose). Some of the guinea pigs were given no treatment (control), the others were given chemotherapy, immunotherapy, or chemotherapy followed by immunotherapy. The median survival of untreated guinea pigs was 56 days. Animals treated with sublethal doses of cyclophosphamide (150 mg/kg) or N,N-bis(2-chlorethyl)-N-nitrosourea (BCNU) 1, 31, or 45 days after tumor cell injection had increased median survival times but were not cured (Table 3). Guinea pigs treated with immunotherapy followed by chemotherapy at the time of peak inflammatory disruption of metastasis, however, survived significantly longer than animals treated with immunotherapy or chemotherapy alone.[52,53]

In each of these treatment groups, some animals were killed on day 45 after tumor inoculation, and their lungs were removed and examined for evidence of macroscopic surface tumor colonies. Guinea pigs treated with immunotherapy followed by chemotherapy had significantly fewer pulmonary tumor foci than did untreated guinea pigs, or guinea pigs given either immunotherapy or chemotherapy alone (Table 4).

These findings suggest that a successful therapeutic approach for metastatic solid tumors might be a process that would both disrupt anatomic barriers and deliver cytotoxic agents to the tumor(s). One host response that could potentially achieve the first goal is an induced cell-mediated hypersensitivity reaction analogous to delayed-cutaneous hypersensitivity occurring at distant (micrometastatic) sites. Thus immune-

Table 3
EFFECT OF COMBINED IMMUNOTHERAPY AND CHEMOTHERAPY ON SURVIVAL OF GUINEA PIGS BEARING LINE 10 TUMORS

Treatment		No. of survivors	%	Comparison with controls (p)	Comparison with animals receiving immunotherapy alone (p)[c]
Immunotherapy[a]	Chemotherapy[b]				
None	None	0/15	0	—	0.042
None	Cyclophosphamide, day 1	0/15	0	—	0.042
None	Cyclophosphamide, day 31	0/15	0	—	0.042
None	BCNU, day 1	0/15	0	—	0.042
Days 10, 17, 24	None	5/15	33	0.042	—
Days 10, 17, 24	Cyclophosphamide, day 31	28/38	74	<0.001	0.011
Days 10, 17, 24	BCNU, day 31	9/15	60	<0.001	0.032
Days 20, 27, 34	Cyclophosphamide, day 10	3/15	20	0.224	0.427
Days 20, 27, 34	None	2/15	13	0.483	0.214

[a]   Immunotherapy was initiated on day 10 or 20 and consisted of three vaccinations spaced 1 week apart. The first two injections contained an admixture of 10^7 BCG and 10^7 line 10 tumor cells. The third injection contained 10^7 line 10 tumor cells alone.

[b]   Chemotherapy was a single i.p. injection of either 150 mg/kg cyclophosphamide or 10 mg/kg BCNU.

[c]   By Fisher's exact test, two-tailed. Pulmonary line-10 tumors were initiated on day 0 by the i.v. injection of 1×10^6 L10 tumor cells.

Table 4
EFFECT OF COMBINED IMMUNOTHERAPY-CHEMOTHERAPY ON THE NUMBER OF PULMONARY TUMOR NODULES IN LINE 10 TUMOR-BEARING GUINEA PIGS

Treatment[a]	Mean number of lung nodules on day 45[b]	Range
None	48 ± 9^c	42—59
Immunotherapy alone	23 ± 7^c	16—29
Chemotherapy alone	26 ± 11^c	14—36
Immunotherapy + chemotherapy	1 ± 2^d	0—4

[a]   All animals received 10^6 L10 tumor cells intravenously on day 0. Animals received no further treatment or were treated with immunotherapy alone beginning on day 10, with cyclophosphamide alone (150 mg/kg) on day 31, or with a combination of immunotherapy and cyclophosphamide chemotherapy

[b]   Animals were killed, and their lungs were fixed for 18 hr in Bouin's solution. The macroscopically observable tumor colonies were counted (n = 3 animals/group).

[c]   Value is significantly different from the untreated group ($p < 0.05$; student's t-test).

[d]   Value is significantly different from all other groups ($p < 0.01$; student's t-test).

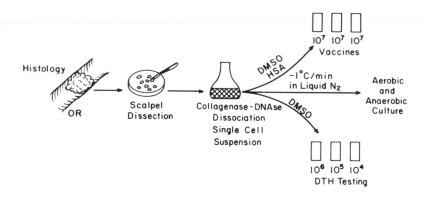

FIGURE 6.   Clinical vaccine development: schema.

mediated hypersensitivity, followed by delivery of blood-borne toxic substances to tumors, could be more effective than either therapy alone.

III. CLINICAL STUDIES OF ACTIVE SPECIFIC IMMUNOTHERAPY

A. A Prospectively Randomized, Controlled Trial of Active Specific Immunotherapy

We translated the results of our experiments with the guinea pig model of active specific immunotherapy into a prospectively randomized, controlled clinical trial of therapy for colorectal cancer in humans 5 years ago.[54-56] There were two questions asked:

1. Can the delayed cutaneous hypersensitivity to autologous tumor cells be boosted by immunotherapy?
2. Can active specific immunotherapy improve the disease-free interval and/or survival when used as an adjuvant to surgery?

In this clinical trial, primary tumors were removed by standard surgical techniques and were enzymatically dissociated and cryopreserved by techniques which maintain cell viability (Figure 6). Adjacent normal colon mucosa was processed similarly. Patients with transmural extension of tumor or nodal metastases were randomized into groups receiving no further treatment or receiving immunotherapy. Skin testing with irradiated, autologous tumor cells and mucosa cells was done 3 weeks postoperatively before immunotherapy began. Immunized patients received one intradermal vaccination weekly for 2 weeks of 10^7 irradiated, autologous tumor cells and 10^7 BCG, and one vaccination of 10^7 irradiated, autologous tumor cells alone in the 3rd week. Skin tests were repeated at 6 weeks, 6 months, and 1 year postvaccination. To date, 47 patients have participated in the trial. The results of this trial show that immunized patients had a significant delayed cutaneous response to their autologous tumor cells (Figure 7). Control patients did not react significantly to tumor or mucosa cells at any test period. In immunized patients, reactivity to tumor cells diminished at 6 months and 1 year but continued to be significantly elevated over control values. Histologic analysis of positive skin test sites revealed marked perivascular infiltrates suggestive of cell-mediated hypersensitivity.

B. Initial Results of the Clinical Trial

With a mean postoperative follow-up period of 36 months there have been 11 recurrences of tumor and 4 deaths in the 25 control patients vs. 5 recurrences and 1 death in the 22 immunized patients.

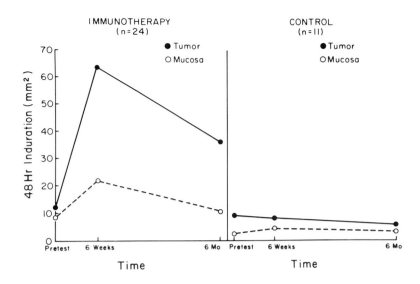

FIGURE 7. Delayed cutaneous hypersensitivity response to tumor and mucosa cell preparations in autologous tumor cell-immunized and nonimmunized patients. The differences between 48-hr induration of tumor and mucosa were statistically significant at 6 weeks ($p < 0.03$) and 6 months ($p < 0.01$) in the treated patients.

Figure 8 depicts each patient's status and shows the site and pathologic stage of the primary tumor and the length of time the patient has been monitored. As expected, most of the recurrences (11 of the 16) were in patients with positive regional lymph nodes. The disease-free status and survival data for patients with positive regional lymph nodes are shown in Figures 9 and 10. Statistical analysis by the one-sided Wilcoxon-Gehan method shows a more significant benefit in both disease-free status ($p = <0.024$) and survival ($p = <0.045$) in this population at higher risk for recurrence and death.

Based on these clinical results and the demonstration in the guinea pig model that there appears to be a synergistic effect between active specific immunotherapy followed by chemotherapy, a phase III prospectively randomized trial of active specific immunotherapy followed by chemotherapy in Dukes' B_2 and C colon cancer patients is underway under the direction of the Eastern Cooperative Oncology Group. This is a multi-institutional study involving 7 clinical centers with an expected accrual of approximately 1000 patients.

Thus, we feel that we have carefully and effectively translated the results of a relevant animal model to the clinic in such a way that the success or failure of active specific immunotherapy as an adjunct to treatment of metastatic diseases of solid tumors will be determined. The results thus far are encouraging. The impact of success in these treatment protocols will be enormous.

IV. CURRENT RESEARCH: GENERATION OF TUMOR CELL-REACTIVE HUMAN MONOCLONAL ANTIBODIES USING PERIPHERAL BLOOD LYMPHOCYTES FROM ACTIVELY IMMUNIZED COLORECTAL PATIENTS

There are three important factors in the development and production of human monoclonal antibodies for TAA. These are strategy, specificity, and stability. Numerous strategies have been attempted over the last few years including the fusion of lymphocytes from lymph nodes draining primary tumors, and Epstein-Barr virus (EBV)

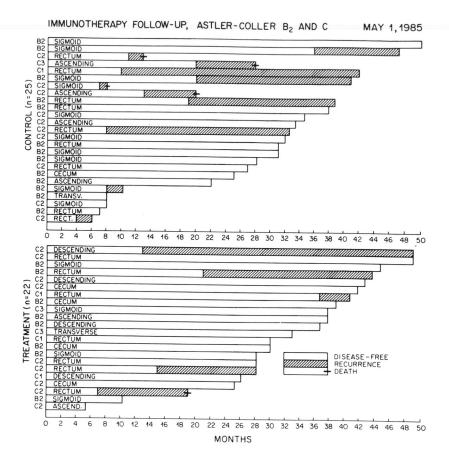

FIGURE 8.   Prospectively randomized trial of adjuvant active specific immunotherapy for human colorectal cancer. Update 5/1/85 (Astler-Coller B and C). Fol-
lowup of all control and immunized patients according to site and pathologic stage.

transformation of peripheral blood lymphocytes and splenocytes from cancer patients.[57-63] Both of these approaches have failed to reproducibly generate human monoclonal antibody reactive with tumor cell surface antigens, presumably because of lack
of immunocompetence of the cancer patient at the time of fusion. Of those hybridomas
produced by these approaches, most only reacted with cytoplasmic antigens, which
made them less valuable from the point of view of in vivo diagnosis and therapy. The
apparent instability of antibody production by EBV-transformed lymphocytes has thus
far made them an impractical means of producing human monoclonal antibody.

We utilized a different approach once we realized that we had, in our phase II active
specific immunotherapy trial, successfully immunized cancer patients to their autochthonous tumor.[64-65] Lymphocytes were obtained from actively immunized patients that
had been determined by delayed cutaneous hypersensitivity tests to be immunologically
responsive to their autologous tumor. In this prospectively randomized protocol, this
induced cell-mediated immune response had been associated with an increase in the
disease-free period and overall survival for patients monitored over 4 years.[55] We spec-
ulated that at some point during the course of immunization, which was developed
primarily for stimulation of a strong cell-mediated immune response, there would be a
transient humoral immune response of some magnitude. In animal models, humoral
immunity is present during the induction of cell-mediated immunity. In our studies the
most productive fusions were obtained with lymphocytes taken 1 week after the first

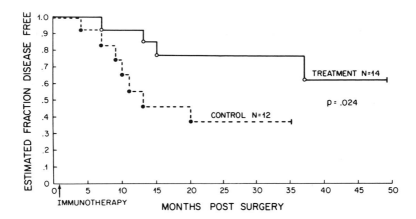

FIGURE 9. Prospectively randomized trial of adjuvant active specific immunotherapy for human colorectal cancer. Disease-free status of all Stage C patients. Update 5/1/85.

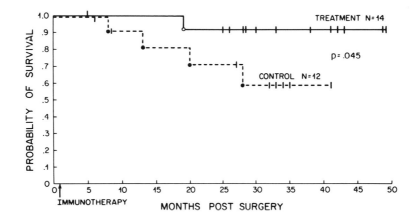

FIGURE 10. Prospectively randomized trial of adjuvant active specific immunotherapy for human colorectal cancer. Survival status of all Stage C patients. Update 5/1/85.

and 1 week after the second immunization (Table 5). In these vaccines, autologous tumor cells were given admixed with BCG at a ratio of 10^7 viable tumor cells to 10^7 viable BCG organisms. Less success in terms of effective fusions was achieved with lymphocytes obtained 1 week after the third immunization, which used the vaccine that consisted solely of tumor cells. No successful fusions with regard to demonstrated production of antibodies reactive with cell surface antigens were obtained in fusions made from patients before immunization. We speculate that the increase in fusion efficiency may be associated with the active immunization augmented by the adjuvant BCG. BCG is known to influence the depletion of bone marrow reserves and thereby to affect the presence of progenitor B-cells in circulation which normally would not be present in the peripheral blood of cancer patients or in lymph nodes draining the sites of primary tumors.

The tissue-reactive human monoclonal antibodies were produced by two cell types distinctly different in morphology and growth pattern. Of the 36 cell lines, 12 were morphologically indistinguishable from murine hybridomas and grew in a dispersed manner. Some six representative cell lines were karyotyped and found to contain both

Table 5

ISOLATION OF HUMAN MONOCLONAL ANTIBODIES REACTIVE WITH
TUMOR CELL SURFACE ANTIGENS

Immu-nization[a]	No. of fusions[b]	No. of wells assayed / No. of wells seeded[c]	No. of Ig+ cell lines[d]	No. of tissue+ MCA[e]	No. of Surface+ MCA / No. of Ig+ cell lines[f]	Isotype[g]		Culture pattern of cell lines[h]	
						IgG	IgM	Diploid	Hybridoma
0	2	25/240 (10)	4	0	0				
1	9	441/1262 (35)	65	10	4/65(6)	2	8	8	2
2	10	573/1688 (34)	154	25	16/154 (10)	9	16	16	9
3	3	112/494 (23)	11	1	0		1		1

[a]   Peripheral blood lymphocytes were obtained 7 days after each immunization except for the preimmunization bleeding.

[b]   Peripheral blood lymphocytes were not available for all time points from the ten patients.

[c]   Wells exhibiting cell growth.

[d]   Production of $\geq 1\ \mu g/m\ell$ human immunoglobulin as measured by a capture enzyme-linked immunosorbent assay (ELISA).

[e]   Immunoperoxidase staining of sections of colorectal tumors.

[f]   Immunoperoxidase staining of nonpermeabilized cultured colon tumor cells or dissociated primary tumor cells, positive reaction on a minimum of two cell lines or dissociated tumors.

[g]   Determined by ELISA.

[h]   Diploid cells grow in large clusters, whereas hybridomas are larger, rounded cells that grow in a dispersed pattern.

murine and human chromosomes. In contrast, most of the tissue-reactive monoclonal antibodies (24 out of 36) were produced by cells that were irregular in shape and grew in large clusters typical of some human lymphoblastoid cell lines. We isolated these cluster-forming cells from seven of ten patients, a result that demonstrates that these cells can be readily isolated when peripheral blood lymphocytes from actively immunized patients are used. The eight cell lines, representing five fusions from four patients, were karyotyped and found to contain, on the average, 46 chromosomes. G-morphology indicated that most of the tumor-reactive monoclonal antibody-synthesizing cell lines were not heterohybridomas, but were transformed B-cells. The 18 representative cluster-forming cells were screened for EBV antigens. All but one of the cell lines were positive for EBNA and only one of the EBNA-positive cell lines was positive for viral capsid antigen.

The individual monoclonal antibodies usually reacted in a homogeneous manner with individual tumors. Rarely did we find a heterogeneous pattern of reactivity among tumor cells, either in paraffin or cryostat sections of an individual tumor with any individual antibody. The pattern of reactivity of 10 of the human monoclonal antibodies to histological sections of colorectal adenocarcinomas from 15 patients is shown in Figure 11. The matrix of reactivity of the antibodies tested indicates that the individual antibodies reacted to between 47 and 80% of the tumor specimens tested. No single antibody reacted to all 15 tumors. In tissue sections from individual patients, the range of reactivity varied from tissues reactive to all ten antibodies (e.g., patients 1, 8, and 11) to tissues reactive to as few as one or two monoclonal antibodies (patients two and nine). All of the tissue specimens used for determination of antibody reactivity were taken from patients other than the ten donors of the B-cells for the original fusions.

We compared the pathologic stage of the tumors tested to the percentage of reactivity with the group of monoclonal antibodies tested and found that the tumors with the broadest reactivity were moderately to well-differentiated adenocarcinomas; the less common, poorly differentiated adenocarcinomas (e.g., patient nine) were generally not

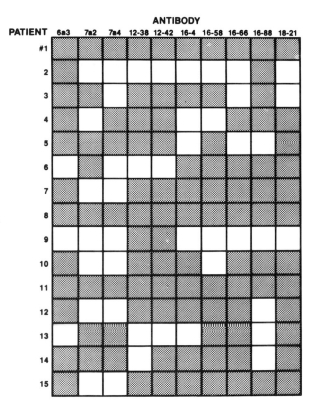

FIGURE 11.   Distribution of antigens in paraffin sections of colorectal tumors.

reactive. The antibodies typically reacted with metastases (e.g., patient four). No pattern of reactivity vis-a-vis site of the primary tumor or Dukes' stage was apparent.

Further direct characterization of the five biotin-labeled monoclonal antibodies with regard to their specificity for tumor vs. normal cells was established with frozen tissue sections of colon tumor and adjacent normal colonic mucosa (Table 6). Absolute specificity was observed in 4 of the antibodies as shown by the fact that they strongly reacted with at least two out of five colon tumors and did not react with any of the four matched normal colonic mucosa sections. Antibody 19b2 reacted strongly with four of five tumor sections and showed a weak reaction with one of four normal colonic mucosa sections.

Frozen sections of normal breast, stomach, kidney, liver, muscle, and skin (Table 6) showed no staining by biotin-labeled human monoclonal antibody except antibody 19b2, which exhibited a low-level of binding to normal stomach tissue. An overall background stain of connective tissue components was observed. This background staining was nonspecific and has been observed by others using biotin-labeled monoclonal antibodies.

To further establish the tumor specificity of the monoclonal antibodies, we tested them for reactivity with carcinoembryonic antigen, human erythrocyte antigens, and human lymphocyte antigens by various techniques. We found no evidence of reaction between these antibodies and these antigens. Reactivity with human erythrocyte antigens was measured by indirect immunofluorescence and hemagglutination against an erythrocyte panel representing all major and most minor blood group systems. No reactivity was seen. Enzyme-linked immunosorbant assay, cytotoxicity assays, and di-

Table 6

REACTIVITY OF BIOTIN-LABELED MONOCLONAL ANTIBODY WITH FROZEN SECTIONS OF COLON TUMORS (T) AND NORMAL TISSUES (N)[a]

Source of tissue	MCA									
	6a3		7a2		7a4		18—22		19b2	
	T	N	T	N	T	N	T	N	T	N
Colon	+	−	−	−	2+	−	+	−	2+	+
Colon	3+	−	2+	−	3+	−	+	−	2+	−
Colon	3+	−	+	−	3+	−	3+	−	3+	−
Colon	2+	−	+	−	−	−	−	−	−	−
Breast	−		−		−		−		−	
Breast	−		−		−		−		−	
Breast	−	−	−	−	−	−	−	−	−	
Stomach	−		−		−		−		+	
Kidney	±[b]		±		±		±		±	
Liver	−		−		−		−		−	
Muscle	−		−		−		−		−	
Skin	−		−		−		−		−	
Skin	−		−		−		−		−	

[a] The presence and degree of binding are indicated as explained in the footnotes to Table 2.

[b] Label limited to cells lining proximal tubules.

rect immunofluorescent staining of human lymphocytes showed no evidence of recognition of human lymphocyte antigens by any of the monoclonal antibodies.

With regard to production, the human monoclonal antibodies were typically produced in the range of 5 to 20 μg/mℓ. No clear differences existed between diploid and hybrid cells in the average quantities of immunoglobulin produced. No murine immunoglobulins were detected in the supernatant fluids of any of the hybrid or diploid cell lines. The diploid cell lines did not exhibit any of the instability reported for lymphoblastoid cell lines obtained by in vitro transformation by EBV. In fact, we observed increases in antibody production with many of the diploid lines during the course of long-term culture. We grew these cells in continuous culture for almost a year without any indication of a finite life span of antibody productivity. Using a single small (25 cc) hollow fiber cartridge, we have been able over the course of 2 months to produce gram quantities of human monoclonal antibodies for two of the cell lines. As expected, the human-mouse heterohybridomas did have a finite, but in most instances, useful life span. Some of the hybrids, as is the case with some mouse-mouse hybrids, were too unstable to be cloned and therefore are not described in this report. Most of the hybrids, however, do appear to have sufficient ability to permit batch production of clinically useful quantities of antibody.

Although stability and specificity is a major consideration in the determination of the usefulness of these tumor-reactive monoclonal antibodies, the lack of reactivity of some of the antibodies to a certain percentage of the tumor specimens is another factor that must be considered. It is unlikely, based upon data obtained with paraffin sections of tumors, dissociated primary tumor cells, and tumor cell lines, that any single monoclonal antibody could react with tumors of all patients, making it ideal for universal therapeutic or diagnostic applications.

The strategy of using immunized cancer patients as a source of PBL has provided a large number of clones from which certain selections can be made in regard to a range

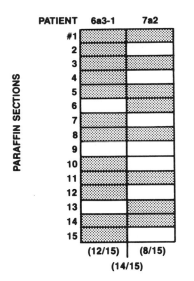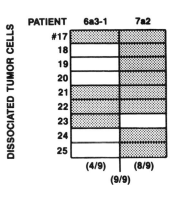

FIGURE 12. Two monoclonal antibodies react with most colorectal tumors.

of reactivities. By selecting only two of the monoclonal antibodies that we have produced which, based on their characteristics in a broad in vitro screen, have the greatest amount of tumor reactivity with the least amount of normal colonic mucosa reactivity, we can propose and develop cocktails of antibodies that together promise greater efficacies than any individual monoclonal antibody. As shown in Figure 12, two monoclonal antibodies paired with a range of reactivity with both tissue sections and dissociated tumor cells and selected based on their relative lack of cross-reactivity with normal colonic mucosa, provide an antibody cocktail which will react with 14 to 15 tumor specimens and 9 of 9 dissociated tumor cell specimens.

V. FUTURE PROSPECTS OF ACTIVE SPECIFIC IMMUNOTHERAPY

Active specific immunotherapy is a therapeutic process that consists of administering a vaccine prepared individually for each patient from the patient's own tumor cells. The strategy for the antitumor usefulness of active specific immunotherapy is the activation of host immune defenses toward antigenic factors unique and distinct for each tumor. Historically, this approach to patient management has been unsuccessful; however, based on optimization of the vaccine conditions in a useful animal model, the technology of active specific immunotherapy has been successfully translated in a randomized phase II clinical study of colorectal cancer. The results of this study demonstrate that clinically significant differences in disease-free intervals and survival can be achieved with active specific immunotherapy. It is important to recognize that this positive and encouraging clinical effect has been achieved in cases of colorectal cancer, a malignancy where no major improvement in treatment has been accomplished in the last two decades. While active specific immunotherapy has had a positive effect, this treatment may not be sufficient for total management of disseminated cancer. Our goal now is to effectively integrate active specific immunotherapy with standard therapeutic modalities and additional forms of biologic therapy. We have demonstrated in the guinea pig model, that there appears to be a synergistic therapeutic effect with active specific immunotherapy followed by chemotherapy. We have recently reported the isolation of more than 30 human monoclonal antibodies reactive with human colorectal carcinoma. These unique reagents, either alone or conjugated with cytotoxic drugs,

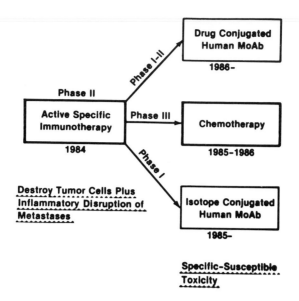

FIGURE 13.   Combinations of biologicals in cancer treatment.

provide the additional armament for multimodal application of specific, nontoxic biologicals in the treatment of solid tumors. Thus, a strategy of active and passive immunotherapy can be anticipated in the management of solid tumors in humans. Our strategy for combinations of biologicals in cancer treatment are shown in Figure 13. Based on the phase II active specific immunotherapy trial in colon cancer, in which the predominant immunologic effect was the destruction of tumor cells plus the inflammatory disruption of metastases, we have translated this trial to a multi-institutional phase III trial combining active specific immunotherapy with chemotherapy. Plans are underway to add adjuvant therapies, including active specific immunotherapy in combination with drug-conjugated human monoclonal antibodies or isotope-conjugated human monoclonal antibodies. Thus, we feel we have the basis for developing rational clinical trials of multimodal therapy using biologicals in a strategic manner. Finally, we recognize the technical limitations of the active specific immunotherapy trials as presently established, which administer a vaccine prepared individually for each patient from the patient's own tumor cells. This is, without question, a procedure that is both labor intensive and technologically complex for the clinical situation. Using the tumor-specific human monoclonal antibodies as probes, we have started the characterization and purification of the reactive antigenic molecules from colon tumor cell lines. Our research goal is the development of an antigenic formulation, or "generic" vaccine, which could ultimately replace the present tumor cell vaccines.

REFERENCES

1. **Gross, L.,** Intradermal immunization of mice against a sarcoma originating in an animal of the same line, *Cancer Res.,* 3, 326, 1943.
2. **Foley, E. J.,** Antigenic properties of methylcholanthrene-induced tumors in mice of the strain of origin, *Cancer Res.,* 13, 35, 1953.
3. **Klein, G.,** Tumor immunology: a general appraisal, in *Scientific Foundation of Oncology,* Symington, T. and Carter, R. L., Eds., Year Book Medical, Chicago, 1976, 497.

4. Hewitt, H. B., Animal tumor models and their relevance to human tumor immunology, *J. Biol. Resp. Modif.,* 1, 107, 1982.

5. Hewitt, H. B., Second point: animal tumor models and their relevance to human tumor immunology, *J. Biol. Resp. Modif.,* 2, 210, 1983.

6. Key, M. E., Brandhorst, J. S., and Hanna, Jr., M. G., More on the relevance of animal tumor models: immunogenicity of transplantable leukemias of recent origin in syngeneic strain 2 guinea pigs, *J. Biol. Resp. Modif.,* 3, 359, 1984.

7. Fujimoto, S., Yamauchi, K., Yamada, S., and Tada, T., Selective stimulation and inactivation of cytotoxic and suppressor T-cells in tumor immunity, in *Immunobiology and Immunotherapy of Cancer,* Terry, W. D. and Yamada, Y., Eds., Elsevier, Amsterdam, 1979, 147.

8. Nind, A. P. P., Nairn, R. C., Pihl, E., Hughes, E. S. R., Cuthbertson, A. M., and Rollo, A. J., Autochthonous humoral and cellular immunoreactivity to colorectal carcinoma: prognostic significance in 400 patients, *Cancer Immunol. Immunother.,* 7, 257, 1980.

9. Werkmeister, J. A., Pihl, E., Nind, A. P. P., Flannery, G. R., and Nairn, R. C., Immunoreactivity by intrinsic lymphoid cells in colorectal carcinoma, *Br. J. Cancer,* 40, 839, 1979.

10. Jubert, A., Talbott, T. M., Mazier, W. P., MacKeigan, J. M., Campos, M. M., Muldoon, J. P., Benjamin, H. E., Ferguson, J. A., and Bowman, H. E., Lymphocyte blastogenic responses to allogeneic leukocytes and autochthonous tumor cells in colorectal carcinoma, *J. Surg. Oncol.,* 9, 171, 1977.

11. Farrar, W. L. and Elgert, K. D., In vitro immune blastogenesis during contact sensitivity in tumor-bearing mice, *Cell. Immunol.,* 40, 365, 1978.

12. Fujimoto, S., Green, M. I., and Sehon, A. H., Regulation of the immune response to tumor antigens. I. Immunosuppressor cells in tumor-bearing hosts, *J. Immunol.,* 116, 791, 1976.

13. Takei, F., Levy, I. G., and Kilburn, D. G., Characterization of suppressor cells in mice bearing syngeneic mastocytoma, *J. Immunol.,* 118, 413, 1977.

14. Treves, A. J., Carnaud, C., Trainin, N., Feldman, M., and Cohen, I. J., Enhancing T lymphocytes from tumor-bearing mice suppresses host resistance to a syngeneic tumor, *Eur. J. Immunol.,* 4, 722, 1974.

15. Yu, A., Watts, H., Jaffe, N., and Parkman, R., Concomitant presence of tumor-specific cytotoxic and inhibitor lymphocytes in patients with osteogenic sarcoma, *N. Engl. J. Med.,* 297, 121, 1977.

16. DeVita, V. T., The relationship between tumor mass and resistance to chemotherapy: implication for surgical adjuvant treatment of cancer, *Cancer,* 51, 1209, 1983.

17. Salmon, S. E. and Jones, S. E., Eds., *Adjuvant Therapy of Cancer,* Vol. 3, Grune & Stratton, New York, 1981.

18. Oldham, R. K. and Smalley, R. V., Immunotherapy: the old and the new, *J. Biol. Resp. Modif.,* 2, 1, 1983.

19. Hanna, M. G., Jr., Zbar, B., and Rapp, H. J., Histopathology of tumor regression following intralesional injection of *Mycobacterium bovis* (BCG). I. Tumor growth and metastasis, *J. Natl. Cancer Inst.,* 48, 1441, 1972.

20. Hanna, M. G., Jr., Zbar, B., and Rapp, H. J., Histopathology of tumor regression following intralesional injection of *Mycobacterium bovis* (BCG). II. Comparative effects of vaccinia virus, oxazolone and turpentine, *J. Natl. Cancer Inst.,* 48, 1697, 1972.

21. Zbar, B., Bernstein, I. D., Bartlett, G. L., Hanna, M. G., Jr., and Rapp, H. J., Immunotherapy of cancer: regression of intradermal tumors and prevention of growth of lymph node metastases after intralesional injection of living *Mycobacterium bovis* (Bacillus Calmette-Guerin), *J. Natl. Cancer Inst.,* 49, 119, 1972.

22. Hanna, M. G., Jr., Snodgrass, M. J., Zbar, B., and Rapp, H. J., Histopathology of tumor regression after intralesional injection of *Mycobacterium bovis.* IV. Development of immunity to tumor cells and to BCG, *J. Natl. Cancer Inst.,* 51, 1897, 1973.

23. Hanna, M. G., Jr. and Peters, L. C., Efficacy of intralesional BCG-therapy in guinea pigs with disseminated tumor, *Cancer,* 36, 1298, 1975..

24. Hanna, M. G., Jr. and Peters, L. C., Immunotherapy of established micrometastases with *Bacillus Calmette-Guerin* tumor cell vaccine, *Cancer Res.,* 38, 204, 1978.

25. Hanna, M. G., Jr. and Peters, L. C., Specific immunotherapy of established visceral micrometastases by BCG-tumor cell vaccine alone or as adjunct to surgery, *Cancer,* 42, 2613, 1978.

26. Hanna, M. G., Jr. and Peters, L. C., BCG immunotherapy: efficacy of BCG-induced tumor immunity in guinea pigs with regional tumor and/or visceral micrometastases, in *Immunotherapy of Human Cancer,* Raven Press, New York, 1978, 111.

27. Peters, L. C., Brandhorst, J. S., and Hanna, M. G., Jr., Preparation of immunotherapeutic autologous tumor cell vaccines from solid tumors, *Cancer Res.,* 39, 1353, 1979.

28. Hanna, M. G., Jr., Active specific immunotherapy of residual micrometastases: a comparison of postoperative treatment with BCG-tumor cell vaccine to preoperative intratumoral BCG injection, in *Immunobiology and Immunotherapy of Cancer,* Terry, W. D. and Yamamura, Y., Eds., Elsevier/North Holland, Amsterdam, 1979, 331.

29. Hanna, M. G., Jr. and Bucana, C., Active specific immunotherapy of residual micrometastases: the acute and chronic inflammatory response in induction of tumor immunity by BCG-tumor cell immunization, *J. Reticuloendothel. Soc.,* 26, 439, 1979.

30. Hanna, M. G., Jr., Brandhorst, J. S., and Peters, L. C., Active specific immunotherapy of residual micrometastasis: an evaluation of sources, doses and ratios of BCG with tumor cells, *Cancer Immunol. Immunother.,* 7, 165, 1979.

31. Hanna, M. G., Jr., Peters, L. C., and Brandhorst, J. S., Active specific immunotherapy of residual micrometastasis: conditions of vaccine preparation and regimen, in *Tumor Progression,* Crispen, R. G., Ed., Elsevier/North Holland, Amsterdam, 1980, 59.

32. Peters, L. C. and Hanna, M. G., Jr., Active specific immunotherapy of established micrometastasis: effect of cryopreservation procedures on tumor cell immunogenicity in guinea pigs, *J. Natl. Cancer Inst.,* 64, 1521, 1980.

33. Hanna, M. G., Jr., Bucana, C. D., and Pollack, V. A., Immunological stimulation *in situ:* the acute and chronic inflammatory responses in the induction of tumor immunity, in *Contemporary Topics in Immunobiology, Vol. 10,* Witz, I. and Hanna, M. G., Jr., Eds., Plenum Press, New York, 1980, 267.

34. Hoover, H. C., Jr., Peters, L. C., Brandhorst, J. S., and Hanna, M. G., Jr., Therapy of spontaneous metastasis with an autologous tumor vaccine in a guinea pig model, *J. Surg. Res.,* 30, 409, 1981.

35. Key, M. E. and Hanna, M. G., Jr., Mechanism of action of BCG-tumor cell vaccines in the generation of systemic tumor immunity. I. Synergism between BCG and line 10 tumor cells in the induction of an inflammatory response, *J. Natl. Cancer Inst.,* 67, 853, 1981.

36. Key, M. E. and Hanna, M. G., Jr., Mechanism of action of BCG-tumor cell vaccines in the generation of systemic tumor immunity. II. Influence of the local inflammatory response on immune reactivity, *J. Natl. Cancer Inst.,* 67, 863, 1981.

37. Hanna, M. G., Jr. and Peters, L. C., Morphological and functional aspects of active specific immunotherapy of established pulmonary metastases in guinea pigs, *Cancer Res.,* 41, 4001, 1981.

38. Key, M. E. and Hanna, M. G., Jr., Antigenic heterogeneity of the guinea pig line 10 hepatocarcinoma. Implications for active specific immunotherapy, *Cancer Immunol. Immunother.,* 12, 211, 1982.

39. Hanna, M. G., Jr., Pollack, V. A., Peters, L. C., and Hoover, H. C., Active specific immunotherapy of established micrometastases with BCG plus tumor cell vaccines: effective treatment of BCG side effects with isoniazid, *Cancer,* 49, 659, 1982.

40. Dvorak, H. F., Dickersin, G. R., Dvorak, A. M., Manseau, E. J., and Pyne, K., Human breast carcinoma: fibrin deposits and desmoplasia. Inflammatory cell-type and distribution. Microvasculature and infection, *J. Natl. Cancer Inst.,* 67, 335, 1981.

41. Dvorak, H. F., Dvorak, A. M., Manseau, E. J., Wiberg, L., and Churchill, W. H., Fibrin gel investment associated with line 1 and line 10 solid tumor growth, angiogenesis, and fibroplasia in guinea pigs. Role of cellular immunity, myofibroblasts, microvascular damage, and infarction in line 1 tumor regression, *J. Natl. Cancer Inst.,* 62, 1459, 1979.

42. Key, M. E. and Haskill, J. S., Immunohistologic evidence for the role of antibody and macrophages in regression of the murine T1699 mammary adenocarcinoma, *Int. J. Cancer,* 28, 225, 1981.

43. Key, M. E., Bernhard, M. I., Hoyer, L. C., Foon, K. A., Oldham, R. K., and Hanna, M. G., Jr., Guinea pig line 10 hepatocarcinoma model for monoclonal antibody serotherapy: *in vivo* localization of a monoclonal antibody in normal and malignant tissues, *J. Immunol.,* 130, 1451, 1983.

44. Haskill, J. S., Key, M. E., Radov, L. A., Parthenais, E., Korn, J. H., Fett, J. W., Yamamura, Y., DeLustro, F., Vesley, J., and Gant, G., The importance of antibody and macrophages in spontaneous and drug-induced regression of the T1699 mammary adenocarcinoma, *J. Reticuloendothel. Soc.,* 26, 417, 1979.

45. Gullino, P. J., Angiogenesis and oncogenesis, *J. Natl. Cancer Inst.,* 61, 639, 1978.

46. West, G. W., Weichselbrum, R., and Little, T. B., Limited penetration of methotrexate into human osteosarcoma spheroids as a proposed model for solid tumor resistance to adjuvant chemotherapy, *Cancer Res.,* 40, 3665, 1980.

47. Hanna, M. G., Jr., Key, M. E., and Oldham, R. K., Biology of cancer therapy: some new insights into adjuvant treatment of metastatic solid tumors, *J. Biol. Resp. Mod.,* 2, 295, 1983.

48. Adelman, N. E., Hammond, M. E., Cohen, S., and Dvorak, H. F., Lymphokines as inflammatory mediators, in *Biology of the lymphokines,* Cohen, S., Pick, E., and Oppenheim, J. J., Eds., Academic Press, New York, 1979, 13.

49. Key, M. E., Bernhard, M. I., Hoyer, L. C., Foon, K. A., Oldham, R. K., and Hanna, M. G., Jr., Guinea pig line 10 hepatocarcinoma model for monoclonal antibody serotherapy. *In vivo* localization of a monoclonal antibody in normal and malignant tissues, *J. Immunol.,* 130, 1451, 1983.

50. Bernhard, M. I., Foon, K. A., Oeltmann, T. N., Key, M. E., Hwang, K. M., Clarke, G. C., Christensen, W. L., Hoyer, L. C., Hanna, M. G., Jr., and Oldham, R. K., Guinea pig line 10 hepatocarcinoma model: characterization of monoclonal antibody and in vivo effect of unconjugated antibody and antibody conjugated to diphtheria toxin A chain, *Cancer Res.,* 43, 4420, 1983.

51. Bernhard, M. I., Hwang, K. M., Foon, K. A., Keenan, A. M., Kessler, R. M., Frincke, J. M., Tallam, D. J., Hanna, M. G., Jr., Peters, L. C., and Oldham, R. K., Localization of ^{111}In- and ^{125}I-labeled monoclonal antibody in guinea pigs bearing line 10 hepatocarcinoma tumors, *Cancer Res.,* 43, 4429, 1983.

52. Hanna, M. G., Jr. and Key, M. E., Immunotherapy of metastases enhances subsequent chemotherapy, *Science,* 217, 367, 1982.

53. Key, M. E., Brandhorst, J. S., and Hanna, M. G., Jr., Synergistic effects of active specific immunotherapy and chemotherapy in guinea pigs with disseminated cancer, *J. Immunol.,* 130, 2987, 1983.

54. Hoover, H. C., Jr., Surdyke, M., Dangel, R. B., Peters, L. C., and Hanna, M. G., Jr., Delayed cutaneous hypersensitivity to autologous tumor cells in colorectal cancer patients immunized with an autologous tumor cell-Bacillus Calmette-Guerin vaccine, *Cancer Res.,* 44, 1671, 1984.

55. Hoover, H. C., Jr., Surdyke, M. G., Dangel, R. B., Peters, L. C., and Hanna, M. G., Jr., Prospectively randomized trial of adjuvant active specific immunotherapy for human colorectal cancer, *Cancer,* 55, 1236, 1985.

56. Hanna, M. G., Jr. and Hoover, H. C., Jr., Active specific immunotherapy as an adjunct to the treatment of metastatic solid tumor, in *Immunity to Cancer,* Academic Press, Orlando, Fla., 1985, (in press).

57. Cole, S. P., Campling, B. G., Louwman, I. H., Kozbor, D., and Roder, J. C., A strategy for the production of human monoclonal antibodies reactive with lung tumor cell lines, *Cancer Res.,* 44, 2750, 1984.

58. Cote, R. J., Morrissey, D. M., Houghton, A. N., Beattie, E. J., Jr., Oettgen, H. F., and Old, L. J., Generation of human monoclonal antibodies reactive with cellular antigens, *Proc. Natl. Acad. Sci. U.S.A.,* 80, 2026, 1983.

59. Cote, R. J., Morrissey, D. M., Oettgen, H. F., and Old, L. J., Analysis of human monoclonal antibodies derived from lymphocytes of patients with cancer, *Fed. Proc.,* 43, 2465, 1984.

60. Iman, A., Drushella, M. M., Taylor, C. R., and Tokes, Z., Generation and immunohistological characterization of human monoclonal antibodies to mammary carcinoma cells, *Cancer Res.,* 45, 263, 1985.

61. Schlom, J., Wunderlich, D., and Teramoto, U. A., Generation of human monoclonal antibodies reactive with human mammary carcinoma cells, *Proc. Natl. Acad. Sci. U.S.A.,* 77, 6841, 1980.

62. Sikora, K., Alderson, T., Ellis, J., Phillips, J., and Watson, J., Human hybridomas from patients with malignant disease, *Br. J. Cancer,* 47, 135, 1983.

63. Sikora, K. and Wright, R., Human monoclonal antibodies to lung-cancer antigens, *Br. J. Cancer,* 43, 696, 1981.

64. Haspel, M. V., McCabe, R. P., Pomato, N., Janesch, N. J., Knowlton, J. V., Peters, L. C., Hoover, H. C., Jr., and Hanna, M. G., Jr., Generation of tumor cell-reactive human monoclonal antibodies using peripheral blood lymphocytes from actively immunized colorectal carcinoma patients, *Cancer Res.,* 45, 3951, 1985.

65. Haspel, M. V., McCabe, R. P., Pomato, N., Hoover, H. C., Jr., and Hanna, M. G., Jr., Human monoclonal antibodies: generation of tumor cell-reactive monoclonal antibodies using peripheral blood lymphocytes from actively immunized colorectal carcinoma patients, in *Monoclonal Antibodies and Cancer Therapy,* Vol. 27, Resifeld, R. A. and Sell, S., Eds., Alan R. Liss, New York, 1985, (in press).

Chapter 13

CURRENT STATUS OF RADIOIMMUNOIMAGING AND THERAPY

Steven M. Larson and Jorge A. Carrasquillo

TABLE OF CONTENTS

I. INTRODUCTION

Monoclonal antibodies[1] against tumor associated antigens[2] may turn out to be extremely effective in the fight against cancer, particularly in regard to the common solid tumors, such as colon, lung, breast, prostate, and ovarian cancers. From the standpoint of Nuclear Medicine, there is already adequate demonstration of the potential for using unique antitumor antibodies for targeting radioactivity to tumors for the dual purposes of diagnosis and therapy (see Figure 1).[3] Reviews have appeared in References 4 and 5. A list of antibodies that have been studied in preliminary clinical trials for either radioimmunoimaging or therapy is shown in Table 1. There are 10 different antitumor antibodies listed from published studies,[6-27] and approximately ten more antitumor antibodies are in various stages of evaluation in patients. Good targeting of radioactivity has been achieved for both hematopoietic and solid tumors. Examples of the clinical research use of antitumor antibodies are shown in Figures 2 and 3. In certain instances, sufficient localization of radioactivity has been achieved to permit consideration of radiotherapy.[28] And yet, despite this promise, there continue to be problems with the degree and reproducibility of localization in tumors. This limits clinical utility of the present methods.[29] If we are to achieve the full potential for the application of antitumor monoclonal antibodies in the fight against cancer, we must overcome certain limitations. These limitations are due to both biologic and technical factors.

II. BIOLOGIC FACTORS LIMITING ANTITUMOR ANTIBODY LOCALIZATION

During the course of the last several years my colleagues and I found evidence that several factors limit the localization of antitumor antibody preparations in human tumors. A listing of the important factors are shown in Table 2. One factor which has not been generally appreciated in nuclear medicine is that the transport of a protein from the blood vascular space into the extracellular fluid is inversely proportional to the molecular weight of the protein.[30] For practical purposes, this can be considered as a barrier to transport of blood-borne antibody into the region of the tumor antigen in the extracellular space. Larger molecular weight immune proteins are most susceptible to this barrier, and smaller molecular weight proteins least susceptible. This may be one reason why Fab fragments are more effective than whole IgG for targeting some types of solid tumors (Figure 4).[31] In the future, we can expect a great deal of development to occur which is directed toward improving the transport of antibody from blood across the capillary barrier into the tumor tissue.

In test tube, the interaction of radiolabeled antibodies and their specific antigen targets follow the chemical laws of mass action. For IgG there are two binding sites, and for Fab fragments, just one binding site. Scatchard analysis[32] has been used to calculate affinities of antibody binding, and the concentration of the antigen present in a reaction mixture. Such considerations underlie the use of specific antibody in immunoassay methods.[33] Basically the many variants of immunoassay quantify the content of antigen based on the magnitude of binding of a labeled antibody/antigen. For example, a mathematical relationship that is often used in a form applicable to actual in vitro binding data in the test tube is as follows:

$$B/F = K[Ag] - K b \qquad (1)$$

where: B is the amount of radiolabeled antibody bound to antigen; F is the free radiolabeled antibody; K is the affinity of binding of the radiolabeled antibody to its

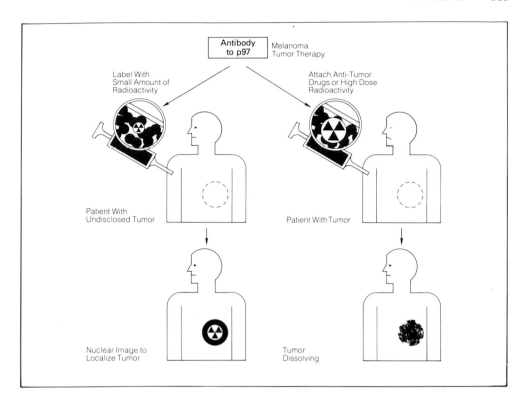

FIGURE 1. Basic principles of radioimmunodetection and radioimmunotherapy. Antibodies as carriers of radioactive tracers for diagnosis and therapy. At low dosage of radioactivity, antibodies are used as tracers; at high dosage of radioactivity, antibodies are used for therapy. The antibody carries the radioactivity to the tumor, and because there are many more antigen sites in tumor than in normal tissues, over time most of the antibody is bound in the tumor in comparison to normal tissues. For diagnostic purposes, a picture of antibody uptake is obtained with a γ-camera. For therapeutic purposes, the radiation deposited in the tumor is enough to selectively damage the tumor. The normal tissues are spared damage because very little radioactivity is retained in these tissues. (From Larson, S. M., *Medicine,* 8, 22, 1981. With permission.)

Table 1
RADIOLABELED MONOCLONAL
ANTIBODIES IN CLINICAL TRIALS

Tumor type	Antibody
Colon	17-1A[6,7,8] 791T36;[9] CEA[10,11] YPC2/12.1[12]
Breast	YPC2/12.1;[12,13] HMFG2[14] LINCRCON-M8;[15] 791T/36[16]
Lung	HMFG2[17]
Ovary	HMFG2;[17,18] 791T/36[19]
Melanoma	96.5;[20 24] 48.7[25]
Sarcoma	791T/36[26]
Lymphoma	T-101[27]

antigen; b is the molar amount of radiolabeled antibody bound to antigen; and [Ag] is the concentration of antigen to which the radiolabeled antibody is binding.

In situations in which the radioactive antibody is in low concentration relative to the concentration of antigen, (antigen excess), the B/F ratio is directly related to the concentration of antigen in the system, and bound to free ratio should increase in a roughly linear way (i.e., since $K b \ll K [Ag]$, equation (1) becomes $B/F = K [Ag]$. In

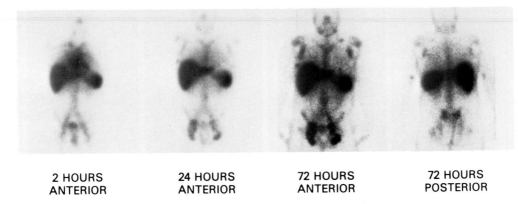

2 HOURS ANTERIOR   **24 HOURS ANTERIOR**   **72 HOURS ANTERIOR**   **72 HOURS POSTERIOR**

FIGURE 2.   Clinical example of targeting of radiolabeled antibody to hematopoietic neoplasm using specific monoclonal antibodies. Serial whole body scans obtained after i.v. injection of 5 mCi (11 mg) of ^{111}In-T101 monoclonal antibody. The patient had biopsy proven cutaneous T-cell lymphoma (CTCL). T-101 antibody binds to an antigen on the cell surface of both malignant and normal T-lymphocytes. The malignant T-lymphocytes express about tenfold greater concentration than normal T-cells. At 2 hr after i.v. injection of the radiolabelled antibody, the radioactivity is still in the blood pool. Significant hepatic and splenic uptake is also seen. By 24 hr after i.v. injection, there is localization in lymph nodes of the pelvis and axilla. By 72 hr, there is even more dense accumulation in the lymph nodes of the cervical area, axilla, retroperitoneal, and inguinal area. In addition there is localization to the skin, where the patient had diffuse erythroderma. Biopsy was performed of the skin and inguinal lymph node. Tumor was documented at these sites. Intravenously administered T-101 targets tumor involvement accurately in CTCL. (From Bunn, P. A., et al., *Lancet*, 1, 1219, 1984. With permission.)

I-131 Fab 96.5 (100 mCi)   OM

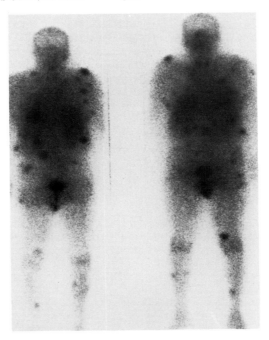

48 hr

FIGURE 3.   Clinical example of targeting of radiolabeled antibody to solid tumor using radiolabeled monoclonal antibodies. Whole body scans obtained at 48 hr after i.v. administration of 100 mCi of ^{131}I on 50 mg of 96.5 Fab fragments. This antibody preparation targets melanoma tumor deposits scattered throughout the body of this patient with disseminated malignant melanoma. The antigen that is recognized is a 97000 dalton mol wt membrane associated glycoprotein. This study was performed as part of a therapeutic trial (NIH), in patients with disseminated melanoma. (From Larson, S. M., *J. Nucl. Med.*, 26, 585, 1985. With permission.)

Table 2
BIOLOGIC FACTORS LIMITING TUMOR LOCALIZATION

Molecular weight of immune protein
Antibody affinity
Antigen content of tumors
Presence of circulating antigen or antimouse antibody in the blood
Cross-reacting antigen on normal tissues
Heterogeneity of antigen expression on tumor deposits
Metabolism of radiolabeled antibody
   Catabolism of antibody
    Removal of radionuclide from antibody
Local tissue factors: capillary permeability; vacularity?

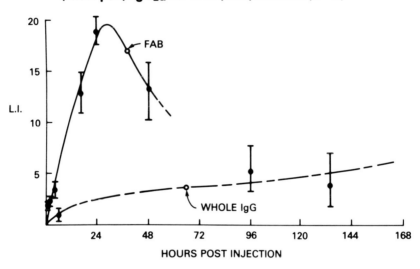

FIGURE 4. Superior targeting of radiolabeled anti-p97 labeled Fab in comparison to IgG in human tumor xenografts. Nude mice received about 80 μg each of IgG or Fab preparations which were labeled with ^{131}I (specific) of ^{125}I (nonspecific), anti-p97 immune proteins. The data is presented as a localization index, which is a measure of the ratio of specific/nonspecific radioactivity, normalized for the blood content. (From Larson, S. M., *J. Nucl. Med.*, 26, 585, 1985. With permission.)

a study that we performed on subjects with metastatic malignant melanoma, subcutaneous nodules were biopsied and the content of the melanoma specific Fab fragment, was compared to a nonspecific control Fab fragment. The ratio of specific to nonspecific, an indicator of the tumor bound/free ratio for radiolabeled antibody, was linearly related to antigen content, as measured by a radioimmunoassay.[22] This is evidence that in vivo, the localization of radiolabeled antibody to tumor is determined in part by the antigen content of tumor in a quantitative binding relationship. When Scatchard plots are used to determine the affinity of antibodies to antitumor antibodies, most antibodies which are clinically useful for targeting of radioactivity in vivo are found to have affinities in the range of 10^8 ℓ/mol to 10^{10} ℓ/mol.

Recent work obtained in nude mice bearing human tumor xenografts provides additional evidence that the in vivo localization of antibody is related to antigen-antibody binding parameters. In a series of tumor xenografts and antitumor antibodies studied at the Wistar Institute (Philadelphia) successful imaging was noted when the product

Table 3
TECHNICAL FACTORS
LIMITING TUMOR
LOCALIZATION

Immunoreactivity of antibody preparations
Bioavailability of radiolabeled antibody
Industrial scale production problems

of the affinity (liter/mole), and the antigen content was greater than a threshold value of 1.5 (when binding sites in 10^6 units were multiplied by affinity in 10^8 ℓ/mol.[34] The importance of the product of the affinity and antigen concentration to determining a target to background ratio that was sufficient for imaging is further evidence that the driving force behind tumor localization is indeed the specific interaction between antibody and antigen.

Other biologic processes, such as capillary transport of antibody, removal of the label from the antibody, catabolism of the antibody, excretion, and clearance into nontumor sites, also influence the degree of localization of radiolabeled antibody in vivo, and the effect of these factors is outside the scope of this review. A brief discussion of the effect of these factors on targeting is described elsewhere.[35]

III. TECHNICAL FACTORS LIMITING ANTITUMOR ANTIBODY LOCALIZATION

A number of technical factors have limited the applicability of radiolabeled antibodies and the most prominent ones are listed in Table 3. In particular, the immunoreactivity of preparations has been a serious limitation in the past. Immunoreactivity can be lost in the labeling process (Figure 5).[36] It can also be lost in the hybridoma stage of monoclonal antibody production, if one member of the fusion pair produces a nonspecific light chain that gets incorporated in some of the monoclonal antibodies. In any event, it is obviously desirable to have 100% of the radiolabeled antibody in an immunoactive form when injected intravenously.

The biologic behavior of the immune preparation can also be altered by improper handling. For example, in addition to the effect on immunoreactivity, the modifications required to label monoclonal antibodies can affect in vivo biodistribution. Thus, most antibodies that have been modified for labeling of metal chelates, such as ^{111}In, tend to concentrate to a greater extent in the liver. This is so prominent in some situations, as to obviate the use of certain products for detecting hepatic metastases.[23,24] There may also be more subtle alterations during the labeling or manufacturing process which cause aggregation or result in nonspecific damage to the radiolabeled antibody. For example, when fragments are used, the digestion processes employed may result in a mixture of IgG, Fab, Fab'$_2$, or smaller fragments. Great care should be taken to ensure that the antibody is in the form desired, and that biologic behavior is intact.

An additional practical problem that has severely limited some clinical research studies, is the difficulty in obtaining gram quantities of well characterized antibodies. New approaches to mass production are currently on the drawing boards or in early operation, however, and we can anticipate that over the next few years the quantities necessary for extensive clinical trials will be available.

IV. COPING STRATEGIES IN RADIOIMMUNODETECTION AND THERAPY

In our experience, each radiolabeled antitumor antibody tends to have its own individual set of characteristics when it comes to in vivo use in humans. For example, some

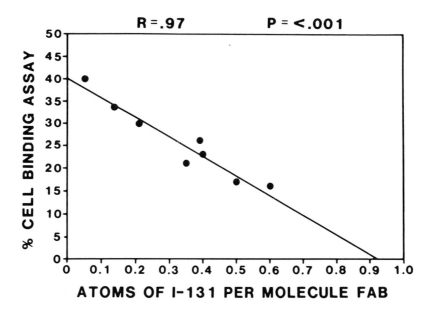

FIGURE 5. Effect of ^{131}I labeling of FAB on cell binding assay. Under the assay conditions, about 40% of the initial radioactivity could be bound to antigen positive cells under conditions in which the radioactivity antibody was labeled at the low specific activity of less than 0.1 atoms of iodine per molecule of FAB. There is an inverse correlation between the retention of immunoreactivity, and the addition of atoms of iodine.[36].

antibodies tend to localize in normal liver, and some do not (e.g., the melanoma antibodies Fab 96.5 and Fab 48.7).[25] When the antibody specificity of the preparation underlies an idiosyncrasy like this, animal models do not predict the result. Thus, in the final analysis, the only way to really learn about a given radiolabeled antibody in detail is to perform clinical research studies in human. Nonetheless, from the experience that we and others have had with radiolabeled antibodies, certain biologic, and technical factors have emerged which limit the localization of the preparation in tumors. We have developed a set of "Coping strategies", which amount to a rough set of guidelines for optimizing the use of these unique antitumor antibodies in the clinical setting (Table 4). These strategies take the known biologic and technical factors into account. Some of these strategies are intuitively obvious, such as pretesting patient subjects to verify the presence of the target antigen in the tumor to be imaged or treated. Other strategies seem to fly in the face of common sense, at least at first impression. For example, when we first proposed that higher doses of antibody mass might actually improve the tumor to surrounding tissue ratio, there was general disbelief. It was thought that the smallest tracer dose of radiolabeled antibody of the highest specific activity should be used, in order to minimize any possibility of saturating tumor associated antigen. Experience has shown that the large antigen content of tumors, and the many competing sites of antibody deposition in vivo, combine to make the optimal dosage size for many radiolabeled antibody preparations to be much larger than previously thought, more nearly in the tens of milligrams range than in the microgram range. In a way this was fortunate, in that relatively low specific activity radiolabeled antibody could be used, that was more likely to be immunoreactive. On the other hand, the requirement for many milligrams per patient has severely taxed the production resources of many investigators, and progress has been slowed by the limited availability of high quality radiolabeled antibody preparations.

Table 4
COPING STRATEGIES IN RADIOIMMUNODETECTION AND THERAPY

Problem	Approach
Large molecular weight immune proteins cross into the tumor ECF very slowly (capillary barrier). This results in low tumor/background tissue ratios	Use Fab's or (Fab'$_2$); Use alternative routes of injection: i.p. or intralymphatic
Many useful antitumor antibodies have sufficient normal tissue cross-reactivity to cause significant uptake in organs such as liver, spleen, lung, or bone marrow	Increasing milligram dose of immune protein will usually improve targeting because tumor antigen concentration is much greater than normal tissue concentration. Normal tissue antigens saturate before tumor antigens (e.g., melanoma)
Not all patients have antigen positive tumors	Prescreen patients with immunohistochemistry tests, and select patients most appropriate for study
There is considerable antigen heterogeneity in vivo from one cancer cell to the next and from one metastatic site to the next	Mixtures of antibodies against different antigens may result in more uniform localization in tumor. However, radiolabeled antibodies may be therapeutically effective on tumor cells many cell diameters away — an advantage for radioimmunotherapy
In certain situations, there is rapid metabolism of the antibody by the tumor cell, with subsequent release of the label. This is likely to be the greatest problem when the antibody antigen complex is internalized, from the cell surface (e.g., T-101 in T-cell lymphomas)	Use a radiolabel, such as ^{111}In or other radiometal, which is not released from the tumor cell
^{111}In-labeled antibodies tend to localize in the normal liver by unknown mechanisms. This obscures metastatic tumor deposits in the liver. Possibly, this phenomenon is due to alterations in the biologic behavior of the immunoglobulin because of the presence of DTPA side chains or damage during the labeling procedure	Use ^{131}I, ^{123}I, or other direct label approach for antitumor antibodies where hepatic metastases are an important consideration. Select optimal dosage or antibody with minimal hepatic cross-reactivity
Immunoreactivity may be lost during labeling resulting in low tumor to tissue ratios. Immunoreactivity tends to be inversely proportional to the number of DTPA's added, or the number of iodine atoms per molecule	Optimize conditions to label at low specific activities. In general, 1 μCi/μg antibody is usually sufficient specific activity. Measure immunoreactivity on each batch of radiolabeled antibody, prior to use
With current preparations of radiolabeled antibodies, tumor to surrounding tissue ratios tend to be low, in the range of 2.5 to 40 to 1. In some instances, especially with deep tumors, of small size, these tumor to surrounding tissue ratios tend to be too small for detection with the planar γ-camera	Utilize *Single Photon Computed Tomography* whenever feasible. The great advantage of this technique is its excellent contrast resolution at depth in tissue
In regard to therapy, penetrating radiation can cause considerable tissue damage away from the site of radiolabeled antibody localization in tumor (e.g., marrow toxicity in the treatment of malignant melanoma with ^{131}I-labeled Fab	Use specialized radiotherapy labels, such as the pure β-emitter, Yt-90, which discharges its energy from a radioactive decay within a few millimeters of the site of localization, and is not associated with any γ-irradiation. For very focal discharge of radiation, within a few cell diameters of decay location, use α-emitters such as Bismuth-212

REFERENCES

1. Kohler, G. and Milstein, C., Continuous culture of fused cells secreting antibody of predefined specificity, *Nature (London)*, 256, 495, 1975.
2. *Genes and Antigens in Cancer Cells: The Monoclonal Antibody Approach*, Vol. 19, S. Karger, Basel, 1984, 121.
3. Larson, S. M., Monoclonal antibodies for diagnosis and therapy: a new frontier in immunology, *Medicine*, 8, 22, 1981.
4. Larson, S. M., Carrasquillo, J. A., and Reynolds, J. C., Radioimmunodetection and radioimmunotherapy, *Cancer Inv.*, 2, 63, 1984.
5. Larson, S. M., Radiolabelled monoclonal anti-tumor antibodies in diagnosis and therapy, *J. Nucl. Med.*, 26, 585, 1985.
6. Chatal, J. F., Detection des tumours par anticorp monoclonaux radiomarquis en tomoscintigraphic, *La Press Med.*, 12, 2361, 1983.
7. Moldofsky, P. J., Powe, J., Mulhern, C. B., Hammond, N., Sears, H. F., Gatenby, R. A., Steplewski, Z., and Koprowski, H., Metastatic colon carcinoma detection with radiolabelled F(ab')$_2$ monoclonal antibody fragments, *Radiology*, 149, 549, 1983.
8. Mach, J-P., Chatal, J-F., Lumbroso, J-D., Bushegger, F., Forni, M., Ritschard, J., Berche, C., Douillard, J. H., Carrel, S., Herlyn, M., Steplewski, Z., and Koprowski, H., Tumor localization in patients by radiolabeled antibodies against colon carcinoma, *Cancer Res.*, 43, 5593, 1983.
9. Farrands, P. A., Pimm, M. V., Embleton, M. J., Perkins, A. C., Hardy, J. D., Baldwin, R. W., and Hardcastle, J. D., Radioimmunodetection of human colorectal cancers by an antitumor monoclonal antibody, *Lancet*, ii, 397, 1982.
10. Mach, J-P., Buchegger, F., Forni, M., et al., Radiolabeled polyclonal and monoclonal antiCEA antibodies for the in vivo detection of human colorectal carcinoma, in *Radioimmunoimaging and Radioimmunotherapy*, Burchiel, S. W. and Rhodes, B. A., Eds., Elsevier Science, Amsterdam, 1983, pp. 345.
11. Mach, J. P., Grob, J. P., Buchegger, F., von Fliedner, V., Carrel, S., Pettavel, J., Bischof-Deloloye, A., and Delaloye, B., Radiolabeled antibodies for the detection of cancer: new approaches to improve the sensitivity and specificity of immunoscintigraphy, *Dev. Oncol.*, 24, 122, 1984.
12. Sikora, K., Smedley, H., and Thorpe, P., Tumor imaging and drug targeting, *Br. Med. Bull.*, 40, 233, 1984.
13. Smedley, H. M., Finan, P., Lennox, E. S., Ritson, A., Takei, F., Wraight, P., and Sikora, K., Localization of metastatic carcinoma by a radiolabeled monoclonal antibody, *Br. J. Cancer*, 47, 253, 1983.
14. Epenetos, A. A., Britton, K. E., Mather, S., et al., Targeting of iodine-123-labeled tumor-associated monoclonal antibodies to ovarian, breast, and gastrointestinal tumors, *Lancet*, 2(8306), 999, 1984.
15. Rainsbury, R. M., Westwood, J. H., Coombes, R. C., Neville, A. M., Ott, R. J., Kalirai, T. S., McCready, V. R., and Gazet, J. C., Location of metastatic breast carcinoma by a monoclonal antibody chelate labeled with indium-11, *Lancet*, 10, 934, 1983.
16. Williams, M. R., Perkins, A. C., Campblee, F. C., Pimm, M. V., Hardy, J. G., Wastie, M. L., Blamey, R. W., and Baldwin, R. W., The use of monoclonal antibody 791T/36 in the immunoscintigraphy of primary and metastatic carcinoma of the breast, *Clin. Oncol.*, 10, 375, 1984.
17. Epenetos, A. A., Courtenay-Luck, N., Halnan, E. I., Hooker, G., Hughes, J. M. B., Krausz, T., Lambert, J., Lavender, J., MacGregor, W. G., McKensie, C. J., Munro, A., Myers, M. J., Orr, J. S., Pearse, E. E., Snook, D., and Webb, B., Antibody guided irradiation of malignant lesions, three cases illustrating a new method of treatment, *Lancet*, 6, 1441, 1984.
18. Epenetos, A. A., Shepherd, J., Britton, K. E., Mather, S., Taylor-Papadimitriou, J., Granowska, M., Durbin, H., Nimmon, C. C., Hawkins, L. R., and Malpas, J. S., ^{123}I-Radioiodinated antibody imaging of occult ovarian cancer, *Cancer*, 55, 984, 1985.
19. Symonds, E. M., Perkins, A. C., Pimm, M. V., Baldwin, R. W., Hardy, J. G., and Williams, D. A., Clinical implications for immunoscintigraphy in patients with ovarian malignancy: a preliminary study using monoclonal antibody 791T/36, *Br. J. Obstet. Gynecol.*, 92, 270, 1985.
20. Larson, S. M., Brown, J. P., Carrasquillo, J. A., et al., Imaging of melanoma with ^{131}I-labeled antibodies, *J. Nucl. Med.*, 24, 123, 1983.
21. Larson, S. M., Carrasquillo, J. A., Krohn, K. A., et al., Diagnostic imaging of malignant melanoma with radiolabeled anit-tumor antibodies, *J. Am. Med. Assoc.*, 249, 811, 1983.
22. Larson, S. M., Carrasquillo, J. A., Krohn, K. A., Brown, J. P., McGuffin, R. W., Fereus, J. M., Graham, M. M., Hill, L. D., Beaumier, P. L., Hellstrom, K. E., and Hellstrom, I., Localization of I-131 labeled p97 specific Fab fragments in human melanoma as a basis for radiotherapy, *J. Cancer Inv.*, 72, 2101, 1983.

23. Murray, J. L., Rosenblum, M. G., Sobol, R. E., Bartholomew, R. M., Plager, C. E., Haynie, T. P., Jahns, M. F., Glenn, H. J., Lamki, L., and Benjamin, R. S., Radioimmunoimaging in malignant melanoma with ¹¹¹In-labeled monoclonal antibody 96.5, *Cancer Res.,* 45, 2376, 1985.
24. Halpern, S. E., Dillman, R. O., Witztum, K. F., Shega, J. F., Hagan, P. L., Burrows, W. M., Dillman, J. B., Clutter, M. L., Sobol, R. E., and Frincke, J. M., Radioimmunodetection of melanoma utilizing In-111 96.5 monoclonal antibody: a prelinimary report, *Radiology,* 155, 493, 1985.
25. Larson, S. M., Carrasquillo, J. A., Krohn, K. A., McGuffin, R. W., Ferens, J. M., Beaumier, P. L., Hellstrom, K. E., and Hellstrom, I., Preliminary clinical experience using and I-131 labeled, murine Fab against a high molecular weight antigen of human melanoma, *Radiology,* 155, 487, 1985.
26. Baldwin, R. W., Embleton, M. J., and Pimm, M. V., Monoclonal antibodies for Radioimmunodetection of tumors and for targeting, *Bull. Cancer (Paris),* 70, 131, 1982.
27. Bunn, P. A., Carrasquillo, J. A., Keenan, A. M., Schroff, R. W., Foon, K. A., Hsu, S-M., Gasdar, A. F., Reynods, J. C., Parentesis, P., and Larson, S. M., Imaging of T-Cell lymphoma by radiolabelled monoclonal antibody, *Lancet,* 11, 1219, 1984.
28. Carrasquillo, J. A., Krohn, K. A., Beaumier, P., McGuffin, R. W., Brown, J. P., Hellstrom, K. E., Hallstrom, I., and Larson, S. M., Diagnosis of and therapy for solid tumors with radiolabelled antibodies and immune fragments, *Cancer Treat. Rep.,* 68, 317, 1984.
29. Mach, J. P., Carrel, S., Forni, M. et al., Tumor localization of radiolabeled antibodies against carcinoembryonic antigen in patients with carcinoma, *N. Engl. J. Med.,* 303, 5, 1980.
30. Nakamura, R. M., Spiegelberg, H., Lee, S., and Weigel, W. O., Relationship between molecular size and intra- and extravascular distribution of protein antigens, *J. Immunol.,* 100, 376, 1968.
31. Beaumier, P. L., Kroh, K. A., Carrasquillo, J. A., Eary, J., Hellstrom, I., Hellstron, K. E., Nelp, W. B., and Larson, S. M., Melanoma localization in nude mice with monoclonal Fab against p97, *J. Nucl. Med.,* 26, 1172, 1985.
32. Scatchard, G., The attraction of proteins for small molecules and ions, *Ann. N. Y. Acad. Sci.,* 51, 660, 1949.
33. Berson, S. A. and Yalow, R. S., Kinetics of reaction between insulin and insulin binding antibody, *J. Clin. Invest.,* 36, 873, 1957.
34. Poise, J., Herlyn, D., Alavi, A., Munz, D., Steplewski, Z., and Koprowski, H., Radioimmunodetection of human tumor xenografts by monoclonal antibodies correlates with antigen density and antibody affinity, in *Immunoscintigraphy,* Britton, K. and Donato, L., Eds., Gordon and Breach, New York, 1985, 139.
35. Larson, S. M., Cancer imaging with monoclonal antibodies, in *Important Advances in Oncology,* DeVita, V. T., Hellman, S., and Rosenberg, S. A., Eds., Lippincott, New York, 1985.
36. Ferens, J. M., Krohn, K. A., Beaumier, P. L., Brown, J. P., Hellstrom, K. E., Carrasquillo, J. A., and Larson, S. M., High-level iodinations of monoclonal antibody fragments for radiotherapy, *J. Nucl. Med.,* 25, 367, 1984.

Chapter 14

THERAPY OF METASTASES BY MONOCLONAL ANTIBODIES AND IMMUNOCONJUGATES

Karl Erik Hellström and Ingegerd Hellström

TABLE OF CONTENTS

I. INTRODUCTION

Monoclonal antibodies have been obtained to many antigens that are expressed more strongly by tumors than by normal tissues and which, with few exceptions, are differentiation antigens.[1-5] Some of these antigens appear to be suitable targets for antibody-based therapy, since they are expressed at high concentrations at the tumor cell surface and are either absent from such cells that are indispensable to the host (e.g., hematopoetic stem cells) or present there at only trace amounts. Both glycoprotein and glycolipid tumor antigens have been identified, and the exact molecular nature is known for several of them. Most of the monoclonal antitumor antibodies have been derived from mice, but a few antibodies of human origin have also been obtained.

We shall discuss here some approaches by which antitumor antibodies can be used therapeutically, alone or as carriers of various agents, such as radioactive isotopes or chemotherapeutic drugs. We have recently reviewed their diagnostic and therapeutic uses, using human melanoma as a model,[4] as well as the use of antibodies for targeting of chemotherapeutic drugs.[5] Therefore, we shall confine this discussion to aspects relating to metastases.

II. ANTIBODY SPECIFICITY FOR TUMOR

If an antibody (or antibody conjugate) is to be used for treatment of tumor metastases, it must be to an antigen whose specificity will allow it to localize to the metastases with some degree of selectivity. The amount of antigen per tumor cell is also important since it must make possible for a sufficient number of molecules of the antibody (conjugate) to bind so that the cell can be destroyed.

Most human tumor antigens defined by monoclonal antibodies are oncofetal or differentiation antigens. This means that they are not only expressed by neoplastic cells but commonly present on normal embryonic cells and, in trace amounts at least, on cells from the normal adult host. Antigen specificity for tumor is, consequently, relative rather than absolute, and is best defined quantitatively as the number of antigen molecules on the neoplastic cells vs. various types of normal cells. Commonly, the neoplastic cells express 10 to 1000 times more of a given antigen than the normal cells with some types of normal cells expressing more than others.[4,6] It is questionable whether any absolutely tumor specific antigens actually exist.[7]

The molecular nature of some tumor antigens has been studied in great detail. For example, a melanoma-associated antigen, p97, has been shown to be a phosphorylated sialoglycoprotein which is structurally homologous to transferrin[8] and coded for by a gene on chromosome 3.[9] cDNA and genomic clones coding for p97 have been obtained, and the whole p97 gene has been sequenced.[10] This forms the basis for transfection studies, development of immunogens ("vaccines"), searches for p97 counterparts in other species, investigations on the regulation of p97 expression in various types of cells, etc. Likewise, the molecular nature of some glycolipid antigens has been characterized in its entirety.[11]

From the detailed information about tumor antigens reached by such studies, it may be possible to find out whether there are any qualitative differences, however small, between antigens expressed in neoplastic as compared to normal cells. There is evidence that a melanoma-associated GD3 antigen has a longer ceramid part than brain GD3.[12] Furthermore, an *O*-acetylated form of GD3 has been identified which has very high specificity for melanoma vs. normal tissues.[13] This probably results from the fact that the expression of this antigen depends on two events, the synthesis of high levels of GD3 antigen and its *O*-acetylation. Either of these events can occur in normal cells but both of them are unlikely to happen in the same normal cell.[13]

It is, of course, possible that antigens of absolute specificity for tumors might be identified with further work. However, the specificity of many of the tumor-associated differentiation antigens already identified probably suffices for therapeutic purposes. As a matter of fact, even antigens that have high expression in certain normal cells might be useful. Thus, idiotypic markers of B-cell lymphomas can be used as targets for therapy,[14] although they are not only shared by the cells of a particular B-lymphoma but also by the clone of normal B-cells from which the lymphoma originated. Antibody targeting of such antigens has given promising results, including one complete, long-lasting remission.[14]

It is common that several differentiation antigens are co-expressed on the same tumor cell while the same normal cell has significant amounts of only one of the antigens. This can be illustrated for melanoma. There are three antigens strongly associated with melanoma: p97,[6,15,16] a proteoglycan,[17-19] and a GD3 ganglioside,[20,21] with most melanomas expressing significant amounts of at least two of the antigens.[22] p97 is present in relatively large amounts on cells from smooth muscle, sweat glands, and liver,[22,23] the proteoglycan is expressed by some endothelial cells,[19] and the GD3 antigen is present on occasional cells in the brain and kidney.[22] On the other hand, few, if any, normal cells have been identified which have significant amounts of more than one of the three antigens. This may be used to develop a strategy for killing melanoma cells expressing at least two of the three antigens while sparing the normal cells. For example, one may use antibody to one antigen to target a molecule to the cell surface which becomes toxic first when combined with a different molecule targeted by antibody to a second antigen.

III. VARIATION IN TUMOR ANTIGEN EXPRESSION

One of the most consistent observations made with tumors is that tumor cell populations display a large amount of variability.[24] This is seen for many different characteristics and includes the expression of tumor antigens.[25,26] If therapy with antibodies is attempted without taking the heterogeneity of antigen expression into account, it may mainly select for antigen-negative cells. Sometimes, evidence for heterogeneity is detectable by immunohistological techniques in that a particular antibody stains some but not all of the neoplastic cells within a tumor nodule. Although some of this heterogeneity may reflect variations dependent on the cell cycle, all antigenic variability cannot be explained this way, since antigen-negative clones can be isolated from originally antigen-positive tumors.[25] Clones lacking one antigen still display other antigens characteristic of the original neoplasm.[25]

To decrease the impact of antigenic heterogeneity on antibody-based therapy, several strategies may be considered. One possibility is to use "cocktails" of antibodies to different antigens,[27] so that cells lacking one antigen can be targeted by an antibody to a second antigen which it still expresses. If antigen-negative variants appear frequently, however, this approach will probably not prevent the emergence of cell clones lacking all the antigens defined by the antibodies in the cocktail. There may, therefore, be a need for targeting of antigen-positive cells in such a way that both these cells and any neighboring antigen-negative tumor cells are destroyed. One way to achieve this may be by labeling the antitumor antibody (cocktail) with a β-particle emitting radioisotope such as ^{131}I, since β-particles can also kill cells at some distance, irrespectively of whether they express the antigen to which the labeled antibody is targeted. Another way may be to so conjugate antibodies with drugs or toxins that free drug (toxin) is released upon contact between the conjugate and antigen-positive cells. There would then be a higher concentration of the therapeutic agent within the tumor than elsewhere in the organism. Third, antibodies may be used for inducing a host reaction at the tumor site, for example, an inflammatory response with activated macrophages, etc., to which neoplastic cells are generally more sensitive than normal cells.[28] Antibodies activating human complement might fit this purpose, as may antibodies coupled with immunomodulating agents, stimulating the activation of either macrophages[28] or NK cells (or both),[29] or inducing so-called LAK cells.[30]

IV. IN VIVO LOCALIZATION OF ANTITUMOR ANTIBODIES

When considering an antitumor antibody for treatment of metastases, it is necessary to ascertain, first, that the metastases express the antigen to which the antibody is directed, and, second, that the antibody (in the form used) can localize to them.

Antibodies binding to a primary tumor but not to its metastases would obviously not be useful for this approach. However, this is unlikely to be the case for most monoclonal antitumor antibodies, since they have been selected for reactivity to metastatic tumors as part of the screening and were often obtained by immunization with metastases. The risk is larger in that some metastases, as a reflection of the heterogeneity of tumor cell populations, lack the antigen to which a given antibody is directed, and that most metastases contain mixtures of antigen-positive and -negative cells, from which the negative cells may be selected (as discussed in Section III).

The next question concerns the ability of an antibody to localize to metastases in vivo. There are two sets of observations relevant in this context. They were made by studying patients with melanoma. These tumors were chosen since they metastasize to many different sites, including the skin, which can easily be biopsied. Mouse antibodies to melanoma cell surface antigens were used in all of the studies.

First, radiolabeled whole antibodies[31,32] or Fab fragments,[33] specific for p97 were shown to localize to human melanomas transplanted to nude mice, while similarly prepared control antibody (Fab) preparations did not, and the ability of a labeled preparation to bind to melanoma cells in vitro was found to correlate with its in vivo localization to tumor.[33] Larson et al.[32,34] then studied human patients using similar antibody preparations. ^{131}I-labeled antibodies specific for p97, or Fab fragments specific for either p97[32,34] or a proteoglycan[35] antigen, were injected intravenously to patients with metastatic melanoma. Tumor uptake could be observed by nuclear imaging as long as the metastases were about 1.5 cm in diameter or larger. This included cutaneous and subcutaneous tumors, as well as tumors in lymph nodes, liver, lung, kidney, and mesenterium.[32,34,35] The immunological specificity of the localization was verified by pair-labeling experiments,[34] in which a selective uptake in tumor biopsies was demonstrated for specific vs. control antibody (Fab fragments). Furthermore, experiments were done in which the same patient was imaged on repeated occasions after having received either ^{131}I-labeled specific Fab fragments, which localized to tumor, or control fragments, which did not.[34]

Second, studies have been performed in which unlabeled antitumor antibodies were given intravenously to melanoma patients. Antibody uptake in skin metastases was verified by immunohistology on biopsies taken at various time points after administration.[36,37] After a patient received approximately 200 mg immunoglobulin (or more), most tumor cells within a metastatic nodule had mouse immunoglobulin bound to their surface, and this was seen throughout the sections. When less than 100 mg of antibody was given, very few cells were stained. Those cells still expressed the respective melanoma antigens, however, since they could be stained by the appropriate antibody in vitro. The results differ from those obtained with antigens which easily undergo antigenic modulation in the presence of antibody. These antigens, as exemplified by the CALLA antigen of leukemic cells, are commonly lost from the cell surface after the cells have been exposed to antibody.[38]

The ability of an antibody (conjugate) to localize to tumors is influenced by many factors, including its molecular size, charge, carbohydrate content, etc. Fab fragments localize more quickly to tumors than whole antibodies,[34] while their lower avidity is a disadvantage. F(ab')₂ fragments may be advantageous both with respect to size and avidity. If an antibody (fragment) is conjugated to another molecule, a drug, for example, this may also to influence its localization to tumor. Various ways to increase this localization should be explored. They might include heating of the tumor area to increase vascular permeability, the use of certain drugs to facilitate the ability of an injected antibody preparation to enter the tumor tissue, induction of inflammation at the tumor site, etc.

V. SOME APPROACHES TO USE ANTITUMOR ANTIBODIES FOR TREATMENT OF METASTASES

A. Antibodies Alone

Antibodies can have an antitumor effect by any of several different mechanisms. First, they can be directly cytolytic or cytostatic, if directed to some molecule that is obligatory to the neoplastic cells or to a receptor mediating the cellular uptake of such a molecule. Antibodies of this type are of particular interest, since they may kill (inhibit) all of a tumor's neoplastic cells, while sparing antigen-negative normal cells. For example, if a given tumor depends on a growth factor that is produced by the tumor cells[39,40] or provided by the host, antibody to this factor or to its receptor may inhibit tumor growth and may even cause tumor destruction. If normal cells are not at all dependent on the factor, or depend on it to a much lesser extent, they may not be harmed.

Antibodies may also be directed to some molecules involved in the invasive growth and metastatic spread of cancer cells. There is a suggestion that antibodies of the latter type exist and may counteract tumor spread in vivo.[41,42]

Furthermore, antibodies may act in consort with either complement or host-cells to kill tumor cells,[43-45] and they may mediate antibody-dependent cellular cytotoxicity (ADCC) in the presence of proper host cells, such as NK cells[45] or macrophages.[46] This may be independent of whether or not the expression of the antigens are defined by the antibody associated with the neoplastic transformation. By activating complement at the tumor site, antibodies may cause an inflammatory reaction with influx of host cells with potential antitumor activity. Sears et al.[46,47] have reported that IgG2a antibodies to an antigen expressed by carcinomas of the colon and pancreas inhibit tumor growth in nude mice by acting in consort with macrophages, and that they may have antitumor activity in some human patients.

Some of the best evidence for tumor cell killing by unmodified antibodies comes from studies on several IgG3 antibodies to a melanoma-associated GD3 antigen. One such antibody, MG-21, has been shown to lyse close to 100% of ⁵¹Cr-labeled melanoma cells in the presence of human complement. It can also mediate ADCC, destroying target cells at an antibody concentration as low as 1 μg/mℓ and a ratio of 1 to 10 leukocytes per target cell; the effector cells are probably related to NK cells, since they express the Leu-11b marker.[45,48] Another anti-GD3 antibody with high ADCC activity, 2B2, was found to inhibit the outgrowth of small (1 × 1 mm) human melanoma transplants in nude mice.[45] Since this may be the size of many micrometastases, a similar ability of the antibody to destroy scattered neoplastic cells in human patients would be expected to be clinically beneficial.

Dramatic antitumor effects of a similar anti-GD3 antibody, R24, have recently been described by Houghton et al. who gave this antibody to patients with metastatic melanoma.[49] Approximately one fourth of the patients had partial responses in the form of regression of both cutaneous and visceral metastases, and several of the remaining patients had evidence for antitumor activity even when it did not qualify as a classical partial response.

In view of the findings obtained, efforts should go into selecting additional antibodies activating human complement and giving ADCC, including antigens expressed by tumors other than melanoma. One approach towards obtaining such antibodies may be by using recombinant DNA technology to splice the gene determining antibody specificity together with a gene determining a desirable biological function.[50-52]

The immunogenicity of repeatedly injected antibodies is a clear problem. It can be decreased by using fragments rather than whole antibodies, and by using human rather than mouse antibodies. The use of "chimeric" (mouse-human) antibodies[50-52] should, for example, decrease this problem. However, even when antibodies that are entirely of human origin are used, their idiotypic and allotypic determinants may still be immunogenic to the treated patients, and procedures for inducing tolerance to those determinants need to be worked out. One should also be aware that there is some evidence that anti-idiotypic antibodies, as they develop in some of the treated patients,[37,53] may have therapeutic benefit.[53]

The quality of antibody preparations (affinity of 10^8 or better, proper isotype, stability, purity) is of crucial importance for all work with either unmodified antibodies or antibodies used as carrier.

B. Radiolabeled Antibodies (Fragments)

Since radiolabeled antibodies and antibody fragments can localize to tumors with some selectivity, it might be possible, by increasing the dose of radioactivity used for labeling, to obtain a therapeutic effect. Encouraging findings using radiolabeled polyclonal antisera have, indeed, been reported by Order who treated patients with hepatoma but often combined the radiolabeled antibodies with other forms of therapy.[54]

A Phase I study was performed on eight patients by Larson's group,[34,35,55] using ^{131}I-labeled Fab fragments specific for either p97 or the melanoma-associated proteoglycan antigen to treat metastatic melanoma. Up to approximately 8000 rads could be delivered to liver metastases with the overall toxicity maintained at an acceptable level, which is encouraging. In one of three patients who received more than 400 mCi ^{131}I, tumor progression was arrested over a 6-month period, and in another patient an i.p. lymph node metastasis regressed.

An advantage of radiolabeled antibodies (fragments) for therapy is that antigen-negative tumor cells can be killed subsequent to the localization of an isotope to antigen-positive cells, as long as the isotope used for labeling has suitable characteristics.[34,56] Another advantage is that one can, by imaging, detect the localization to tumor of the agent used to treat it. Furthermore, even if the dose of radiation to tumor which can be safely obtained only increases by a factor of 2 to 3, this may have significant therapeutic benefit. There are also disadvantages in using radiolabeled antibodies for therapy, however. Radiation damage may occur to sensitive tissues, such as bone marrow and gut, even when these tissues express very little of the target antigen; this can follow from both immunologically nonspecific uptake of antibodies (fragments) and secondary radiation from antibodies localizing to tumor.[34,56] Furthermore, treatment of large patient groups with radiolabeled antibodies would pose logistical problems in view of the need to isolate the patients for several days after treatment.

C. Drug (Toxin) Conjugates

Antibodies can be conjugated to toxins[57,58] or drugs[59-62] and become selectively cytotoxic to antigen-positive cells. If this does not impair their localization to tumors, selective damage to neoplastic vs. normal tissues may be obtained. Even if a conjugate gives only a three to five times better localization to tumor than to normal tissues, this may be sufficient to affect a cure of certain tumors.

Conjugates have been made between some toxins and antibodies, and found to be selectively cytotoxic to antigen-positive tumor cells in vitro.[57,58,63,64] Their in vivo effects have been less impressive, however, although antitumor responses have been observed with some conjugates given to animals with transplanted tumors.[58,64] So far, toxin conjugates have not been much tested in human cancer patients.

Likewise, conjugates have been made between antibodies and various anticancer drugs. One of the more encouraging observations comes from a study by Tsukada et al.[65] Antibodies to alphafetoprotein (AFP) were conjugated with daunamycin and used to treat rats with an ascites hepatoma which expressed AFP at the cell surface. When the conjugate was injected intravenously to the rats, significant antitumor activity was observed. This included several cures.

There are two potential problems with drug-antibody conjugates which must be considered. First, if cancer cells are not able to take up the conjugated drug, there may be no therapeutic benefit. Conjugates binding to antigens which easily undergo antigenic modulation[66] may be the ones easily taken up by cells. When the target antigens do not modulate in the presence of antibody, some techniques may be needed for improving conjugate uptake, e.g., via endocytosis, or to cause the release of free-drug upon contact with the tumor. It is important to realize, however, that anti-p97 conjugates with either ricin (A-chain[63]) or vindesine[62] were found to have high antitumor activity in vitro in spite of the fact that p97 does not modulate.[67]

Second, there is a risk that treatment with a conjugate will just select for antigen-negative tumor cells. This is in view of the fact that tumor cell populations are heterogeneous with antigen losses known to occur. The use of antibody cocktails or conjugates releasing the anticancer drug upon contact with antigen-positive cells might decrease the impact of this problem as discussed in Section III.

Conjugates between antibodies (antibody fragments) and tumor inhibiting molecules such as interferon, tumor necrosis factor,[68] various tumor growth inhibitor factors,[69] or molecules inducing differentiation,[70] should also be considered, in view of the possibility that such conjugates may have high selectivity for cancer cells. Furthermore, conjugates with immunomodulating drugs or lymphokines may offer therapeutic advantages, since they, too, may affect neoplastic cells much more than their normal counterparts, by inducing a host response to which the cancer cells are more sensitive. Encouraging results in the treatment of lung and liver metastases, have been obtained in animal systems, using either activated macrophages[28] or "LAK cells",[30] the latter given in combination with IL-2. If antibodies could be used to target such cells to tumors, therapeutic effects may be achieved with little toxicity.

Various combinations of unconjugated antibodies, chemotherapeutic drugs, drug conjugates, and biological response modifiers such as interferon or IL-2 should, of course, also be considered.

D. Active Immunization

Active immunization has some advantages over passive antibody therapy, as exemplified in the combat of infectious diseases. It would, for example, be attractive, if procedures could be developed for inducing a tumoricidal host response in cancer patients, which destroys those small numbers of tumor cells which remain after conventional therapy and which can counteract, over a long period of time, the emergence of additional tumor cells.

For this reason one may, after a tumor antigen has been identified by a monoclonal antibody, attempt to develop some form of active immunization. As immunogen for this, one may use either the antigen[71] or an anti-idiotypic antibody.[72-82] The antigen may be derived from a patient's own neoplastic cells or come from some other source. For example, peptide antigens may be synthesized and protein antigens obtained via recombinant DNA technology[10] and various glycolipid antigens can be prepared. Anti-idiotypic antibodies using a monoclonal antibody as the immunogen can be obtained in the form of polyclonal sera but probably better as monoclonal anti-idiotypic antibodies. These may act as "internal images" of the antigens, or, in some other way, up-regulate a tumoricidal host response to the tumor.[82]

Before the use of active immunogens should be tried in patients, two questions need to be answered. First, is it, indeed, possible to induce an immune response to tumor-associated differentiation antigens, since these may appear as "self" to the immune system of the host? Second, if this can be done, will the immune response damage normal tissues, expressing a small amount of the given antigens? These questions could be studied in model systems which are available.[83,84] We expect the first question to be answered affirmatively. This is in view of recent experiments, in which anti-idiotypic antibody related to a mouse bladder carcinoma antigen was shown to induce cell-mediated tumor immunity in vivo,[85] in spite of the fact that the bladder tumor antigen was expressed on normal embryonic cells and, in trace amounts, on some normal adult mouse cells.[84,85] It remains unclear, however, whether an immunity so induced can cause tumor destruction in vivo and whether it will have an adverse affect on normal tissues.

If it would prove feasible to induce a tumoricidal immune response to tumor-associated antigens, without unacceptable side-effects on normal tissues, the patient, following removal of a primary tumor, may be immunized in such a way that any remaining metastatic cells are killed. However, in view of the heterogeneity of tumor cell populations, this approach will probably work only if its target is a molecule that plays a key role in the neoplastic transformation, or if the immune response succeeds in destroying also those tumor cell variants that lack the antigen to which the response was induced. If the "vaccination" procedure can activate macrophages or NK cells or induce LAK cells, at all sites of metastatic tumor, the latter might be achieved.

VI. CONCLUSIONS

Monoclonal antibodies, alone, labeled with radioisotope, or conjugated with drug, toxin, or biological response modifier, may be used to target and destroy metastatic tumor cells. "Vaccines" in the form of anti-idiotypic antibodies or tumor antigen, developed after an antigen has been first defined by monoclonal antibody, may also be considered, since they might be employed to induce active tumor immunity. The problem of tumor cell heterogeneity is perhaps the largest one to overcome for any of these forms of therapy to be successful. It may call for a therapeutic approach in which antigen-positive cells are used to target to a tumor therapeutic agents which can also destroy antigen-negative tumor cells.

ACKNOWLEDGMENT

The work of the authors has been supported by grants CA 38011, CA 39211, and CA 29639 from the National Cancer Institute, and by support from ONCOGEN. The authors want to acknowledge collaborative work with Paul L. Beaumier, Joseph P. Brown, and Steven M. Larson. The secretarial assistance of Mrs. Phyllis Harps is gratefully acknowledged.

REFERENCES

1. Reisfeld, R. A. and Ferrone, S., Eds., *Melanoma Antigens and Antibodies,* Plenus Press, New York, 1982.
2. Riethmuller, G., Koprowski, H., von Kleist, S., and Munk, K., Eds., *Contributions to Oncology,* Vol. 19, S. Karger, Basel, 1984.
3. Baldwin, R. W. and Byers, V. S., Eds., *Monoclonal Antibodies for Tumor Detection and Drug Targeting,* Academic Press, in press.
4. Hellström, I. and Hellström, K. E., Clinical potential of monoclonal antibodies as studied with human melanoma, in *Accomplishments in Cancer Research,* Fortner, J. F. and Rhoads, J. E., Eds., Lippincott, New York, 1985, 216.
5. Hellström, K. E., Hellström, I., and Goodman, G. E., Antibodies for drug delivery, in *Sustained and Controlled Release Drug Delivery Systems,* Robinson, J. R. and Lee, V. H. L., Eds., Marcel Dekker, New York, in press.
6. Brown, J. P., Nishiyama, K., Hellström, I., Hellström, K. E., Structural characterization of human melanoma-associated antigen p97 using monoclonal antibodies, *J. Immunol.,* 127, 539, 1981.
7. Bageshaw, K. D., Tumour markers — where do we go from here?, *Br. J. Cancer,* 48, 167, 1983.
8. Brown, J. P., Hewick, R. M., Hellström, I., Hellström, K. E., Doolittle, R. F., and Dreyer, W. J., Human melanoma-associated antigen p97 is structurally and functionally related to transferrin, *Nature (London),* 296, 171, 1982.
9. Plowman, G. D., Brown, J. P., Enns, C. A., Schroder, J., Nikinmaa, B., H. H., Hellström, K. E., and Hellström, I., Assignment of the gene for human melanoma-associated antigen p97 to chromosome 3, *Nature (London),* 303, 70, 1983.
10. Rose, T. M., Plowman, G. D., Teplow, D. B., Dreyer, W. J., Hellström, K. E., and Brown, J. P., Primary structure of the human melanoma antigen p97 (melanotransferrin) deduced from the mRNA sequence, *Proc. Natl. Acad. Sci. U.S.A.,* 83, 1261, 1986.
11. Hakomori, S., Tumor associated carbohydrate antigens, *Ann. Rev., Immunol.,* 2, 103, 1984.
12. Nudelman, E., Hakomori, S., Kannagi, R., Levery, S., Yeh, M.-Y., Hellström, K. E., and Hellström, I., Characterization of a human melanoma-associated ganglioside antigen defined by a monoclonal antibody, *J. Biol. Chem.,* 257, 12752, 1982.
13. Cheresh, D. A. and Reisfeld, R. A., O-Acetylation of disialoganglioside GD3 by human melanoma cells creates a unique antigenic determinant, *Science,* 225, 844, 1984.
14. Miller, R. A., Maloney, D. G., Warnke, R., Levy, R., Treatment of B-cell lymphoma with monoclonal anti-idiotypice antibody, *N. Engl. J. Med.,* 306, 517, 1981.
15. Woodbury, R. G., Brown, J. P., Loop, S. M., Hellström, K. E., Hellström, I., Identification of a cell surface protein, p97, in human melanomas and certain other neoplasms, *Proc. Natl. Acad. Sci. U.S.A.,* 77, 2183, 1980.
16. Brown, J. P., Woodbury, R. G., Hart, C. E., Hellström, I., and Hellström, K. E., Quantitative analysis of melanoma-associated antigen p97 in normal and neoplastic tissues, *Proc. Natl. Acad. Sci. U.S.A.,* 78, 539, 1981.
17. Bumol, T. F. and Reisfeld, R. A., Unique glycoprotein-proteoglycan complex defined by monoclonal antibody on human melanoma cells, *Proc. Natl. Acad. Sci. U.S.A.,* 79, 1245, 1982.
18. Ferrone, S., Giacomini, P., Natali, P. G., Ruiter, D., Buraggi, L., Callegaro, L., and Rose, U., A high molecular weight-melanoma associated antigen (HWM-MAA) defined by monoclonal antibodies: a useful marker to radioimage tumor lesions in patients with melanoma, in *Proc. 1st Int. Symp. Neutron Capture Ther.,* Fairchild, R. G. and Brownell, G. L., Eds., Brookhaven National Laboratories, La Crosse, Wis., 1983, 174.
19. Hellström, I., Garrigues, H. J., Cabasco, L., Mosely, G. H., Brown, J. P., and Hellström, K. E., Studies of a high molecular weight human melanoma-associated antigen, *J. Immunol.,* 130, 1467, 1983.
20. Dippold, W. G., Lloyd, K. O., Li, L. T. C., Ikeda, H., Oettgen, H. F., and Old, L. J., Cell surface antigens of human malignant melanoma: definition of six antigenic systems with mouse monoclonal antibodies, *Proc. Natl. Acad. Sci. U.S.A.,* 77, 6114, 1980.
21. Yeh, M.-Y., Hellström, I., Abe, K., Hakomori, S., and Hellström, K. E., A cell surface antigen which is present in the ganglioside fraction and shared by human melanomas, *Int. J. Cancer,* 29, 269, 1982.
22. Hellström, K. E., Hellström, I., Brown, J. P., Larson, S. M., Nepom, G. T., and Carrasquillo, J. A., Three human melanoma-associated antigens and their possible clinical application, in *Contributions to Oncology,* Vol. 19, Riethmuller, G., Koprowski, H., von Kleist, S., and Munk, K., Eds., S. Karger, Basel, 1984, 121.
23. Garrigues, H. J., Tilgen, W., Hellström, I., Franke, W., and Hellström, K. E., Detection of a human melanoma-associated antigen, p97, in histological sections of primary human melanomas, *Int. J. Cancer,* 29, 511, 1982.

24. Foulds, L., Progression and carcinogenesis, *Acta Un-Int Cancer,* 17, 148, 1961.

25. Yeh, M.-Y., Hellstrom, I., and Hellstrom, K. E., Clonal variation in expression of a human melanoma antigen defined by a monoclonal antibody, *J. Immunol.,* 126, 1312, 1981.

26. Albino, A. P., Lloyd, K. O., Houghton, A. N., Oettgen, H. F., and Old, L. J., Heterogeneity in surface antigen and glycoprotein expression of cell lines derived from different melanoma metastases of the same patient, *J. Exp. Med.,* 154, 1764, 1981.

27. Natali, P. G., Bigotti, A., Cavaliere, R., Liao, S.-K., Taniguichi, M., Matsui, M., and Ferrone, S., Heterogeneous expression of melanoma-associated antigens and HLA antigens by primary and multiple metastatic lesions removed from patients with melanoma, *Cancer Res.,* 45, 2883, 1985.

28. Fidler, I. J. and Poste, G., Macrophage-mediated destruction of malignant tumor cells and new strategies for the therapy of metastatic disease, *Springer Semin. Immunopathol.,* 5, 161, 1982.

29. Herberman, R. B., Ed., *Natural Cell-Mediated Immunity Against Tumors,* Academic Press, New York, 1980.

30. Mule, J. J., Shu, S., Schwartz, S. L., and Rosenberg, S. A., Adoptive immunotherapy of established pulmonary metastases with LAK cells and recombinant interleukin-2, *Science,* 1984, 225, 1487.

31. Matzku, S., Mattern, J., George, P., and Hellström, I., Radioimmunolocalization of melanomas with monoclonal antibodies directed against the p97 marker: model experiments in vitro and in nude mice bearing transplanted human melanomas, in *Gasteiner Interantionales Symposium,* Egermann, Ed., Verlag, 1982, 295.

32. Larson, S. M., Brown, J. P., Wright, P. W., Carrasquillo, J. A., Hellström, I., and Hellström, K. E., Imaging of melanoma with ^{131}I-labelled monoclonal antibodies, *J. Nucl. Med.,* 24, 123, 1983.

33. Beaumier, P., Krohn, K., Carrasquillo, J., Eary, J., Hellström, K. E., Hellström, I., Nelp, W., and Larson, W., Melanoma localization in nude mice with monoclonal Fab against p97, *J. Nucl. Med.,* in press.

34. Larson, S. M., Carrasquillo, J. A., Krohn, K. A., Brown, J. P., McGuffin, R. W., Ferens, J. M., Graham, M. M., Hill, L. D., Beaumier, P. L., Hellström, K. E., and Hellström, I., Localization of p97 specific Fab fragments in human melanoma as a basis for radiotherapy, *J. Clin. Invest.,* 72, 2101, 1983.

35. Larson, S. M., Carrasquillo, J. A., McGuffin, R. W., Krohn, K. A., Ferens, J. M., Hill, L. D., Beaumier, P. L., Hellström, K. E., and Hellström, I., Preliminary clinical experiments using ^{131}I-labelled murine Fab against a high molecular weight antigen of human melanoma, *Radiology,* 155, 487, 1985.

36. Oldham, R. K., Foon, K. A., Morgan, A. C., Woodhouse, C. S., Schraff, R. S., Abrams, P. G., Fer, M., Schoenberg, C. S., Farrell, M., Kimball, E., and Sherwin, S. A., Monoclonal antibody therapy of malignant melanoma: in vivo localization in cutaneous metastasis after intravenous administration, *J. Clin. Oncol.,* 2, 1935, 1984.

37. Goodman, G. E., Beaumier, P. L., Hellström, I., Fernyhough, B., and Hellström, K. E., Phase I trial of murine monoclonal antibodies in patients with advanced melanoma, *J. Clin. Oncol.,* 3, 340, 1985.

38. Ritz, J., Pesando, U. J. M., and Sallan, S. E., Serotherapy of acute lymphoblastic leukemia with monoclonal antibody, *Blood,* 58, 141, 1981.

39. Todaro, G. J., Marquardt, H., Twardzik, D. R., Reynolds, F. H., Jr., and Stephenson, J. R., Transforming growth factors produced by viral-transformed and human tumor cells, in *Biological Responses in Cancer: Progress Toward Potential Applications,* Vol. 2., Mihich, E., Ed., Plenum Press, New York, 1984, 1.

40. Marquardt, H., Hunkapiller, M. W., Hood, L. E., and Todaro, G. J., Rat transforming growth factor — 1. Structure and relation to epidermal growth, *Science,* 223, 1079, 1984.

41. Vollmers, H. P. and Birchmeier, W., Monoclonal antibodies inhibit the adhesion of mouse B16 melanoma cells in vitro and block lung metastases in vivo, *Proc. Natl. Acad. Sci. U.S.A.,* 80, 3729, 1983.

42. Vollmers, H. P. and Birchmeier, W., Monoclonal antibodies that prevent adhesion of B16 melanoma cells and reduce metastases in mice: cross-reaction with human tumor cells, *Proc. Natl. Acad. Sci. U.S.A.,* 80, 6863, 1983.

43. Yeh, M.-Y., Hellström, I., Brown, J. P., Warner, G. A., Hansen, J. A., and Hellström, K. E., Cell surface antigens of human melanoma identified by monoclonal antibody, *Proc. Natl. Acad. Sci. U.S.A.,* 76, 2927, 1979.

44. Hellström, I., Brown, J. P., and Hellström, K. E., Monoclonal antibodies to two determinants of melanoma-antigen p97 act synergistically in complement-dependent cytotoxicity, *J. Immunol.,* 127, 157, 1981.

45. Hellström, I., Brankovan, V., and Hellström, K. E., IgG3 antibodies to a human melanoma-associated ganglioside antigen with strong antitumor activities, *Proc. Natl. Acad. Sci. U.S.A.,* 82, 1499, 1985.

46. Sears, H. F., Mattis, J., Herlyn, D., Hayry, P., Atkinson, B., Ernst, C., Steplewski, Z., and Koprowski, H., Phase I clinical trial of monoclonal antibody in treatment of gastrointestinal tumors, *Lancet,* 1, 762, 1982.

47. Sears, H. F., Herlyn, D., Koprowski, H., and Wen Shen, J., Immunotherapy of gastrointestinal malignancies with a murein IgG2a antibody, in *Contributions to Oncology,* Vol. 19, Riethmuller, G., Koprowski, H., van Kliest, S., and Munk, K., S. Karger, Basel, 1984, 180.

48. Hellström, K. E., Hellström, I., Goodman, G. E., and Brankovan, V., Antibody-dependent cellular cytotoxicity to human melanoma antigens, in *Monoclonal Antibodies and Cancer Therapy,* Vol. 27, Reisfeld, R. A. and Sell, S., Alan R. Liss, New York, 1985, in press.

49. Houghton, A. N., Mintzer, D., Cordon-Cardo, C., Welt, S., Fliegel, B., Vadham, S., Carswell, E., Melamed, M. R., Oettgen, H. F., and Old, L. J., Mouse monoclonal IgG3 antibody detecting GD3 ganglioside — a phase I trial in patients with malignant melanoma, *Proc. Natl. Acad. Sci. U.S.A.,* 82, 1242, 1985.

50. Morrison, S. L., Johnson, M. J., Herzenberg, L. A., and Oi, V. T., Chimeric human antibodies molecules: mouse antigen-binding domains with human constant region domains, *Proc. Natl. Acad. Sci. U.S.A.,* 81, 6851, 1984.

51. Neuberger, M. S., Williams, G. T., and Fox, R. O., Recombinant antibodies possessing novel effector functions, *Nature (London),* 312, 604, 1984.

52. Takeda, S., Naito, T., Hama, K., Noma, T., and Honjo, T., Construction of chimaeric processed immunoglobulin genes containing mouse variable and human constant region sequences, *Nature (London),* 314, 452, 1985.

53. Koprowski, H., Herlyn, D., Lubeck, M., DeFreitas, E., and Sears, H. F., Human antiidiotype antibodies in cancer patients: is the modulation of the immune response beneficial for the patient?, *Proc. Natl. Acad. Sci. U.S.A.,* 81, 216, 1984.

54. Order, S. E., Radioimmunoglobulin therapy of cancer, *Compr. Ther.,* 10, 9, 1984.

55. Carrasquillo, J. A., Krohn, K. A., Beaumier, P., McGuffin, R. W., Brown, J. P., Hellström, K. E., Hellström, I., and Larson, S. M., Diagnosis and therapy of solid tumors with radiolabelled Fab, *Cancer Treat. Rep.,* 68, 317, 1984.

56. DeNardo, G. L., Raventos, A., Hines, H. H., Scheibe, P. O., Macey, D. J., Hays, M. T., and DeNardo, S. J., Requirements for a treatment planning system for radioimmunotherapy, *Int. J. Radiat. Oncol. Biol. Phys.,* 11, 335, 1985.

57. Jansen, F. K., Blythman, H. E., Carriere, D., Casellas, P., Gros, O., Gros, P., Laurent, J. C., Paolucci, F., Pau, B., Poncelet, P., Richer, G., Vidal, H., and Voisin, G. A., Immunotoxins: hybrid molecules combining high specificity and potent cytotoxicity, *Immunol. Rev.,* 62, 185, 1982.

58. Vitetta, E. S. and Uhr, J. W., The potential use of immunotoxins in transplantation, cancer therapy, and immunoregulation, *Transplantation,* 37, 535, 1984.

59. Mathe, G., Loc, T. B., and Bernard, J., Medecine Experimetale — Effet sur la leucemia 1210 de la Souris d'une combinaison par diazotation d'A-methopterine et de y-globuines de hamsters porteurs de celle leucemia par heterogreffe, *C. R. Acad. Sci.,* 246, 1626, 1958.

60. Ghose, T., Norvell, S. T., Guclu, A., Cameron, D., Bodurtha, A., and MacDonald, A. S., Immunochemotherapy of cancer with chlorambucil-carrying antibody, *Br. Med. J.,* 3, 495, 1972.

61. Hurwitz, R., Levy, R., Maron, R., Wilchek, M., Arnon, R., and Sela, M., The covalent binding of daunomycin and adriamycin to antibodies, *Cancer Res.,* 35, 1175, 1975.

62. Rowland, G. F., Axtan, C. A., Baldwin, R. W., Brown, J. P., Corvalan, J. R. F., Embleton, M. J., Gore, V. A., Hellström, I., Hellström, K. E., Jacobs, E., Marsdan, C. H., Pimm, M. V., Simmonds, R. G., and Smith, W., Antitumor properties of vindesine-monoclonal antibody conjugates, *Cancer Immunol. Immunother.,* 19, 1, 1985.

63. Casellas, P., Brown, J. P., Gros, O., Gros, P., Hellström, I., Jansen, F. K., Poncelet, P., Vidal, H., and Hellström, K. E., Human melanoma cells can be killed in vitro by an immunotoxin specific for melanoma-associated antigen p97, *Int. J. Cancer,* 30, 437, 1982.

64. Bumol, T. F., Wang, Q. C., Reisfeld, R. A., and Kaplan, N. O., Monoclonal antibody and antibody-toxin conjugate to a cell surface proteoglycan, *Proc. Natl. Acad. Sci. U.S.A.,* 80, 529, 1983.

65. Tsukada, I., Bishop, W. K., Hibe, N., Hirai, E., Hurwitz, E., and Sela, M., Effect of conjugates of daunomycin and antibodies to rat alphafeto-protein-producing tumor cells, *Proc. Natl. Acad. Sci. U.S.A.,* 79, 621, 1982.

66. Old, L. J., Stockert, E., Boyse, E. A., and Kim, J. H., Antigen modulation: loss of TL antigen from cells exposed to TL antibody. Study of the phenomenon in vitro, *J. Exp. Med.,* 127, 523, 1968.

67. Hellström, I., Brown, J. P., and Hellström, K. E., Melanoma-associated antigen p97 continues to be expressed after prolonged exposure of cells to specific antibody, *Int. J. Cancer,* 31, 553, 1983.

68. Carswell, E. A., Old, L. J., Kassel, R. L., Green, S., Fiore, N., and Williamson, B., An endotoxin-induced serum factor that causes necrosis of tumors, *Proc. Natl. Acad. Sci. U.S.A.,* 72, 3666, 1975.

69. Fryling, C. M., Iwata, K. K., Johnson, P. A., Knott, W. B., and Todaro, G. J., Two distinct tumor cell growth-inhibiting factors from a human rhabdomyosarcoma cell lines, *Cancer Res.*, 45, 2695, 1985.

70. Meyskens, F. J., Jr., Gilmartin, E., Alberts, D. S., Levine, R., Brooks, S. E., and Surwit, E. A., Activity of isoretinoin against squamous cell cancers and pre-neoplastic lesions, *Cancer Treat. Rep.*, 66, 1315, 1982.

71. Atassi, M. Z., Precise determination of the entire antigenic structure of lysozyme: molecular features of protein antigenic structures and potential of surface stimulation systhesis — a powerful new concept for protein binding sites, *Immunochemistry*, 15, 909, 1978.

72. Jerne, N. K., The immune system: a web of V domains, *Harvey Lect.*, 70, 93, 1975.

73. Rajewski, K. and Takemori, T., Genetics, expression, and function of idotypes, *Ann. Rev. Immunol.*, 1, 569, 1983.

74. Binz, H. and Wigzell, H., Shared idiotypic determinants on B and T lymphocytes reactive against the same antigenic determinants. III. Physical fractionation of specific immunocompetent T lymphocytes by affinity chromatography using anti-idiotypic antibodies, *J. Exp. Med.*, 142, 1231, 1975.

75. Hedrick, S. M., Nielson, E. A., Kavaler, J., Cohen, D. I., and Davis, M. M., Isolation of cDNA clones encoding T cell specific membrane associated proteins, *Nature (London)*, 308, 149, 1984.

76. Bluestone, J. A., Sharrow, S. O., Epstein, S. L., Ozato, K., and Sachs, D. H., Induction of anti-h-2 antibodies without alloantigen exposure by in vivo administration of anti-idiotype, *Nature (London)*, 291, 233, 1981.

77. Ertl, H., Greene, M., Noseworthy, J., Fields, B., Nepom, J. T., Spriggs, D., and Finburg, R., Identification of idiotypic receptors on reovirus specific cytolytic T cells, *Proc. Natl. Acad. Sci. U.S.A.*, 79, 7479, 1982.

78. Kennedy, R. C., Melnick, J. L., and Dreesman, G. R., Antibody to hepatitis, B virus induced by injecting antibodies to the idiotype, *Science*, 223, 930, 1984.

79. Binz, H., Meier, B., and Wigzell, H., Induction or elimination of tumor-specific immunity against a chemically induced rat tumor using auto-anti-idiotypic antibodies, *Int. J. Cancer*, 29, 417, 1982.

80. Forstrom, J. W., Nelson, K. A., Nepom, G. T., Hellström, I., and Hellström, K. E., Immunization to a syngeneic sarcoma by a monoclonal autoantiidiotypic antibody, *Nature (London)*, 303, 627, 1983.

81. Nelson, K. A., Hellström, I., and Hellström, K. E., Tumor antigen-specific suppressor factors made by T cell hybridomas, in *T-Cell Hybridomas*, Taussig, M. J., Ed., CRC Press, Boca Raton, Fla., 1985, 129.

82. Nepom, G. T., Nelson, K. A., Holbeck, S. L., Hellström, I., and Hellström, K. E., Induction of immunity to a human tumor marker by in vivo administration of anti-idiotypic antibodies in mice, *Proc. Natl. Acad. Sci. U.S.A.*, 81, 2864, 1984.

83. Hellström, I., Rollins, N., Settle, S., Chapman, P., Chapman, W. H., and Hellström, K. E., Monoclonal antibodies to two mouse bladder carcinoma antigens, *Int. J. Cancer*, 29, 175, 1982.

84. Hellström, I., Hellström, K. E., Rollins, N., Lee, V. K., Hudkins, K., and Nepom, G. T., Monoclonal antibodies to cell surface antigens shared by chemically induced mouse bladder carcinoma, *Cancer Res.*, 45, 2210, 1985.

85. Lee, V. K., Harriott, T. G., Kuchroo, V. K., Halliday, W. J., Hellström, I., and Hellström, K. E., Monoclonal anti-idiotypic antibodies related to a murine oncofetal bladder tumor antigen induce specific cell-mediated tumor immunity, *Proc. Natl. Acad. Sci. U.S.A.*, 82, 6286, 1985.

86. Hellström, I., Unpublished observation

INDEX